BC Cancer Agency
CARE & RESEARCH

While the BC Cancer Agency considers this information to be useful, it may vary from our standard practice and protocol.

It is intended for educational purposes only and should not be substituted for the advice of a healthcare professional.

Green Tea

FOOD SCIENCE AND TECHNOLOGY

A Series of Monographs, Textbooks, and Reference Books

1. Flavor Research: Principles and Techniques, *R. Teranishi, I. Hornstein, P. Issenberg, and E. L. Wick*
2. Principles of Enzymology for the Food Sciences, *John R. Whitaker*
3. Low-Temperature Preservation of Foods and Living Matter, *Owen R. Fennema, William D. Powrie, and Elmer H. Marth*
4. Principles of Food Science
   Part I: Food Chemistry, *edited by Owen R. Fennema*
   Part II: Physical Methods of Food Preservation, *Marcus Karel, Owen R. Fennema, and Daryl B. Lund*
5. Food Emulsions, *edited by Stig E. Friberg*
6. Nutritional and Safety Aspects of Food Processing, *edited by Steven R. Tannenbaum*
7. Flavor Research: Recent Advances, *edited by R. Teranishi, Robert A. Flath, and Hiroshi Sugisawa*
8. Computer-Aided Techniques in Food Technology, *edited by Israel Saguy*
9. Handbook of Tropical Foods, *edited by Harvey T. Chan*
10. Antimicrobials in Foods, *edited by Alfred Larry Branen and P. Michael Davidson*

11. Food Constituents and Food Residues: Their Chromatographic Determination, *edited by James F. Lawrence*
12. Aspartame: Physiology and Biochemistry, *edited by Lewis D. Stegink and L. J. Filer, Jr.*
13. Handbook of Vitamins: Nutritional, Biochemical, and Clinical Aspects, *edited by Lawrence J. Machlin*
14. Starch Conversion Technology, *edited by G. M. A. van Beynum and J. A. Roels*
15. Food Chemistry: Second Edition, Revised and Expanded, *edited by Owen R. Fennema*
16. Sensory Evaluation of Food: Statistical Methods and Procedures, *Michael O'Mahony*
17. Alternative Sweeteners, *edited by Lyn O'Brien Nabors and Robert C. Gelardi*
18. Citrus Fruits and Their Products: Analysis and Technology, *S. V. Ting and Russell L. Rouseff*
19. Engineering Properties of Foods, *edited by M. A. Rao and S. S. H. Rizvi*
20. Umami: A Basic Taste, *edited by Yojiro Kawamura and Morley R. Kare*
21. Food Biotechnology, *edited by Dietrich Knorr*
22. Food Texture: Instrumental and Sensory Measurement, *edited by Howard R. Moskowitz*
23. Seafoods and Fish Oils in Human Health and Disease, *John E. Kinsella*
24. Postharvest Physiology of Vegetables, *edited by J. Weichmann*
25. Handbook of Dietary Fiber: An Applied Approach, *Mark L. Dreher*
26. Food Toxicology, Parts A and B, *Jose M. Concon*
27. Modern Carbohydrate Chemistry, *Roger W. Binkley*
28. Trace Minerals in Foods, *edited by Kenneth T. Smith*
29. Protein Quality and the Effects of Processing, *edited by R. Dixon Phillips and John W. Finley*
30. Adulteration of Fruit Juice Beverages, *edited by Steven Nagy, John A. Attaway, and Martha E. Rhodes*
31. Foodborne Bacterial Pathogens, *edited by Michael P. Doyle*
32. Legumes: Chemistry, Technology, and Human Nutrition, *edited by Ruth H. Matthews*
33. Industrialization of Indigenous Fermented Foods, *edited by Keith H. Steinkraus*
34. International Food Regulation Handbook: Policy • Science • Law, *edited by Roger D. Middlekauff and Philippe Shubik*
35. Food Additives, *edited by A. Larry Branen, P. Michael Davidson, and Seppo Salminen*
36. Safety of Irradiated Foods, *J. F. Diehl*
37. Omega-3 Fatty Acids in Health and Disease, *edited by Robert S. Lees and Marcus Karel*
38. Food Emulsions: Second Edition, Revised and Expanded, *edited by Kåre Larsson and Stig E. Friberg*
39. Seafood: Effects of Technology on Nutrition, *George M. Pigott and Barbee W. Tucker*
40. Handbook of Vitamins: Second Edition, Revised and Expanded, *edited by Lawrence J. Machlin*

41. Handbook of Cereal Science and Technology, *Klaus J. Lorenz and Karel Kulp*
42. Food Processing Operations and Scale-Up, *Kenneth J. Valentas, Leon Levine, and J. Peter Clark*
43. Fish Quality Control by Computer Vision, *edited by L. F. Pau and R. Olafsson*
44. Volatile Compounds in Foods and Beverages, *edited by Henk Maarse*
45. Instrumental Methods for Quality Assurance in Foods, *edited by Daniel Y. C. Fung and Richard F. Matthews*
46. *Listeria*, Listeriosis, and Food Safety, *Elliot T. Ryser and Elmer H. Marth*
47. Acesulfame-K, *edited by D. G. Mayer and F. H. Kemper*
48. Alternative Sweeteners: Second Edition, Revised and Expanded, *edited by Lyn O'Brien Nabors and Robert C. Gelardi*
49. Food Extrusion Science and Technology, *edited by Jozef L. Kokini, Chi-Tang Ho, and Mukund V. Karwe*
50. Surimi Technology, *edited by Tyre C. Lanier and Chong M. Lee*
51. Handbook of Food Engineering, *edited by Dennis R. Heldman and Daryl B. Lund*
52. Food Analysis by HPLC, *edited by Leo M. L. Nollet*
53. Fatty Acids in Foods and Their Health Implications, *edited by Ching Kuang Chow*
54. *Clostridium botulinum*: Ecology and Control in Foods, *edited by Andreas H. W. Hauschild and Karen L. Dodds*
55. Cereals in Breadmaking: A Molecular Colloidal Approach, *Ann-Charlotte Eliasson and Kåre Larsson*
56. Low-Calorie Foods Handbook, *edited by Aaron M. Altschul*
57. Antimicrobials in Foods: Second Edition, Revised and Expanded, *edited by P. Michael Davidson and Alfred Larry Branen*
58. Lactic Acid Bacteria, *edited by Seppo Salminen and Atte von Wright*
59. Rice Science and Technology, *edited by Wayne E. Marshall and James I. Wadsworth*
60. Food Biosensor Analysis, *edited by Gabriele Wagner and George G. Guilbault*
61. Principles of Enzymology for the Food Sciences: Second Edition, *John R. Whitaker*
62. Carbohydrate Polyesters as Fat Substitutes, *edited by Casimir C. Akoh and Barry G. Swanson*
63. Engineering Properties of Foods: Second Edition, Revised and Expanded, *edited by M. A. Rao and S. S. H. Rizvi*
64. Handbook of Brewing, *edited by William A. Hardwick*
65. Analyzing Food for Nutrition Labeling and Hazardous Contaminants, *edited by Ike J. Jeon and William G. Ikins*
66. Ingredient Interactions: Effects on Food Quality, *edited by Anilkumar G. Gaonkar*
67. Food Polysaccharides and Their Applications, *edited by Alistair M. Stephen*
68. Safety of Irradiated Foods: Second Edition, Revised and Expanded, *J. F. Diehl*
69. Nutrition Labeling Handbook, *edited by Ralph Shapiro*

70. Handbook of Fruit Science and Technology: Production, Composition, Storage, and Processing, *edited by D. K. Salunkhe and S. S. Kadam*
71. Food Antioxidants: Technological, Toxicological, and Health Perspectives, *edited by D. L. Madhavi, S. S. Deshpande, and D. K. Salunkhe*
72. Freezing Effects on Food Quality, *edited by Lester E. Jeremiah*
73. Handbook of Indigenous Fermented Foods: Second Edition, Revised and Expanded, *edited by Keith H. Steinkraus*
74. Carbohydrates in Food, *edited by Ann-Charlotte Eliasson*
75. Baked Goods Freshness: Technology, Evaluation, and Inhibition of Staling, *edited by Ronald E. Hebeda and Henry F. Zobel*
76. Food Chemistry: Third Edition, *edited by Owen R. Fennema*
77. Handbook of Food Analysis: Volumes 1 and 2, *edited by Leo M. L. Nollet*
78. Computerized Control Systems in the Food Industry, *edited by Gauri S. Mittal*
79. Techniques for Analyzing Food Aroma, *edited by Ray Marsili*
80. Food Proteins and Their Applications, *edited by Srinivasan Damodaran and Alain Paraf*
81. Food Emulsions: Third Edition, Revised and Expanded, *edited by Stig E. Friberg and Kåre Larsson*
82. Nonthermal Preservation of Foods, *Gustavo V. Barbosa-Cánovas, Usha R. Pothakamury, Enrique Palou, and Barry G. Swanson*
83. Milk and Dairy Product Technology, *Edgar Spreer*
84. Applied Dairy Microbiology, *edited by Elmer H. Marth and James L. Steele*
85. Lactic Acid Bacteria: Microbiology and Functional Aspects: Second Edition, Revised and Expanded, *edited by Seppo Salminen and Atte von Wright*
86. Handbook of Vegetable Science and Technology: Production, Composition, Storage, and Processing, *edited by D. K. Salunkhe and S. S. Kadam*
87. Polysaccharide Association Structures in Food, *edited by Reginald H. Walter*
88. Food Lipids: Chemistry, Nutrition, and Biotechnology, *edited by Casimir C. Akoh and David B. Min*
89. Spice Science and Technology, *Kenji Hirasa and Mitsuo Takemasa*
90. Dairy Technology: Principles of Milk Properties and Processes, *P. Walstra, T. J. Geurts, A. Noomen, A. Jellema, and M. A. J. S. van Boekel*
91. Coloring of Food, Drugs, and Cosmetics, *Gisbert Otterstätter*
92. *Listeria*, Listeriosis, and Food Safety: Second Edition, Revised and Expanded, *edited by Elliot T. Ryser and Elmer H. Marth*
93. Complex Carbohydrates in Foods, *edited by Susan Sungsoo Cho, Leon Prosky, and Mark Dreher*
94. Handbook of Food Preservation, *edited by M. Shafiur Rahman*
95. International Food Safety Handbook: Science, International Regulation, and Control, *edited by Kees van der Heijden, Maged Younes, Lawrence Fishbein, and Sanford Miller*
96. Fatty Acids in Foods and Their Health Implications: Second Edition, Revised and Expanded, *edited by Ching Kuang Chow*

Additional Volumes in Preparation

Green Tea

Health Benefits and Applications

Yukihiko Hara

Tokyo Food Techno Co., Ltd.
(Mitsui Norin Co., Ltd.)
Tokyo, Japan

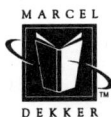

MARCEL DEKKER, INC.   NEW YORK · BASEL

DEKKER

Library of Congress Cataloging-in-Publication Data

Green tea : health benefits and applications / Yukihiko Hara.
    p. cm. — (Food science and technology ; 106)
Includes index.
ISBN 0-8247-0470-3 (alk. paper)
    1. Green tea—Health aspects. I. Title. II. Food science and technology
(Marcel Dekker, Inc.) ; 106.

RM240.H37 2000
615'.323624—dc21

00-047597
CIP

This book is printed on acid-free paper.

Headquarters
Marcel Dekker, Inc.
270 Madison Avenue, New York, NY 10016
tel: 212-696-9000; fax: 212-685-4540

Eastern Hemisphere Distribution
Marcel Dekker AG
Hutgasse 4, Postfach 812, CH-4001 Basel, Switzerland
tel: 41-61-261-8482; fax: 41-61-261-8896

World Wide Web
http://www.dekker.com

The publisher offers discounts on this book when ordered in bulk quantities. For more information, write to Special Sales/Professional Marketing at the headquarters address above.

Current printing (last digit):
10 9 8 7 6 5 4 3 2 1

PRINTED IN THE UNITED STATES OF AMERICA

Foreword

What you eat and drink can be the cause of a disabling or deadly disease, or it can extend your life span to a healthy old age. What is beneficial and what is harmful? In the United States, and many other countries, investments have been made in medical research that have led to major successes in disease prevention, diagnosis, and therapy. Advances in the basic sciences such as nutrition, biochemistry, pharmacology, and pathology have provided an understanding of cell and tissue behavior and factors that impinge on their proper functioning, as well as the elements that go wrong and lead to disease processes.

Despite these advances, however, there is still significant premature mortality from cardiovascular diseases, many types of cancer, and problems associated with aging, such as Alzheimer's disease and other mental and psychiatric conditions. Many of these diseases have been found to be associated with nutritional traditions, eating habits, and life-style. For example, cigarette smoking is a cause of sudden heart attacks and cancers of the lung, pancreas, kidney, bladder, and cervix worldwide. Smokers also have a higher risk of emphysema. Tobacco chewing or snuff dipping leads to cancer of the mouth and esophagus. Excessive alcohol use potentiates the effect of tobacco, and by itself causes cancer of the esophagus and rectum, as well as diseases of the liver, including cirrhosis. It may also increase the risk of breast cancer. In the Western world, about 30% of premature mortality is seen in tobacco users. There are considerable international efforts to control the use of tobacco, especially of cigarette smoking. Tobacco farming and taxes on tobacco provide revenues to governments, but this income is small compared to the high cost of diagnosing and treating the disease associated with tobacco use.

On the other hand, some foods and beverages have a protective effect. This statement is based on national and, especially, on international differences in disease incidence as a function of locally prevailing nutritional habits. At the present time, coronary heart disease is a major problem in much of the West, but cerebrovascular diseases and stroke occur frequently in Asia and, in particular, in Japan and parts of China. People in the Western world suffer from cancer of the breast, colon, prostate, ovary, and endometrium (uterus), whereas in the Far East these cancers have a low incidence, but cancer of the stomach and esophagus are major problems. In Africa, there are areas with endemic cancer of the liver, and in Egypt and other countries bordering the Nile River, cancer of the urinary bladder is frequent.

International, coordinated research has provided leads or, in many instances, factual information on the causes of these major diseases as a sound basis for recommendations for prevention through avoidance of these causes. Smoking and tobacco use have already been cited as risk factors for certain diseases; it is also known that populations with a high sodium intake have a risk of stroke and gastric cancer. Populations with a high total fat intake have a risk of nutritionally linked cancers, such as those in the colon, breast, and prostate. Yet, not all fats have the same adverse effects. Olive oil and canola oil do not increase the risk of the nutritionally linked cancers and of heart disease. There is a lower incidence of heart disease and the nutritionally linked cancers in the Mediterranean region, in particular in Greece and southern Italy, where olive oil is favored. Nevertheless, digestible oils or fats have the same high caloric value of 7 kcal/g, compared to only 4 kcal/g for starches and proteins. This high caloric value needs to be taken into account to avoid obesity, a major problem in North America. Obesity stems from excessive caloric intake over calorie needs for the normal functioning of the body. Populations of industrialized nations tend to be more and more sedentary, with the consequent lower caloric requirement.

Wholesome drinking water supplies are also important. Most people in the Western world, in Japan, and in most regions of the large subcontinent of China have access to running water that is treated through filtration and chlorination to be safe to drink. Regrettably, in some areas of the world, water is contaminated by bacteria and undesirable chemicals. One solution to avoid bacterial contamination is to boil the water before use. The introduction of the wholesome and tasty beverage of tea thousands of years ago has provided a universal solution to the problem of providing humanity with a safe beverage. However, there are many additional benefits to the intake of tea. First, adults should consume about 2–2.5 liters of fluids a day. About one-third—700–800 ml—might be in the form of hot or cold tea. In the Orient, green tea is favored, but in most of the Western world, black tea is the beverage of choice.

Tea comes from the top leaves of the plant *Camellia sinensis*. These leaves contain as principal product a powerful antioxidant, epigallocatechin gallate (EGCg), and minor amounts of other catechins. All these chemicals are polyphenols. The fresh leaves also contain an enzyme, polyphenol oxidase. When the freshly collected leaves are treated with steam or heated in a pan, the polyphenol oxidase is inactivated. Drying of the heated leaves followed by chopping and rolling yields

green tea. If upon harvest and chopping to liberate the polyphenol oxidase the leaves are allowed to stand at about 40°C
for 30 minutes, there is a partial biochemical oxidation of the
polyphenols and the result is oolong tea, favored in southern
China and Southeast Asia. Allowing the oxidation to run for
60–90 minutes converts the polyphenols to those typical of
black tea, such as theaflavins and thearubigins.

Detailed research shows that the antioxidant polyphenols from green, oolong, or black tea have similar beneficial
effects. For example, they decrease the oxidation of LDL-
cholesterol, a risk factor for coronary heart disease. The antioxidants also reduce the oxidation of DNA, consequent to the
action of carcinogens and to the peroxidation reactions on lipids, generating oxy radicals and peroxides. In addition, they
can induce enzymes in tissues such as liver that help detoxify
harmful chemicals, including carcinogens, and lower the risk
of promoting chemicals in the overall cancer process. Tea
polyphenols also decrease the rate of cell duplication, especially of abnormal, transformed cells involved in cancer development. This property slows the growth of early cancer cells
and may even be beneficial as adjuvant therapy of neoplasia.
There are also some indications that regular intake of tea
modifies the intestinal bacterial flora, enhancing the growth
of beneficial bacteria and eliminating those with possibly
harmful attributes. Clearly, tea is an inexpensive beverage,
that is easily made, hot or cold, and pleasant and tasty. It can
be consumed neat or with a little milk, sugar, or lemon. It is
sterile regardless of the quality of water used, since boiling is
the customary way of preparing it.

The scientific progress in the field of tea and health has
been remarkable in the past 15 years. These advances have
been recorded in numerous scientific publications, reviews,
and presentations at symposia and conferences. Yet, a single
overview of the many aspects of tea production, its inherent
properties and constituents, analysis, chemical and biochemical functions, actions in lowering risk of cardiovascular diseases and cancers, and the relevant underlying mechanisms

has not been available. We owe a debt to Dr. Yukihiko Hara for providing a detailed treatise on this topic that particularly emphasizes the significant health benefits to be gained by the oral intake of tea catechins. In addition, his discussion of their practical utility is sure to be of interest not only to those in tea and health sectors but also in other diverse industries where possibilities for utilizing tea catechins exist. Dr. Hara is one of the world's experts on the manifold aspects of tea and health, and we are indebted to him for taking the time to enrich us by sharing his vast knowledge.

John H. Weisburger, Ph.D., M.D.
American Health Foundation
Valhalla, New York

Preface

The importance of research on tea and health has been well recognized worldwide since around 1990, and several international symposiums in succession have been held on this theme. The first, "Tea Quality-Human Health," was held in Hanzhou, China, in 1987, followed by the "International Symposium on Tea Science" in Shizuoka, Japan (1991). "Tea and Human Health," organized by Dr. John H. Weisburger of the American Health Foundation, Valhalla, New York, was also held in 1991. Those interested in the physiological aspects of tea were invited to this symposium, and I had the privilege to attend it.

This book deals primarily with the health benefits of tea polyphenols—in particular, of tea catechins, which are the major components in fresh tea leaves and are responsible for the pungency of green tea. Tea polyphenols, via oral intake or topical application, work miraculously in maintaining good

health and fighting against the deterioration or aggravation
of age-related or life-style-related malconditions to which we
are all prone.

Tea is a refreshing, thirst-quenching beverage. Moreover,
the benefits of tea drinking on human health have long been
taught by generations of people who in their daily lives used
tea as a home remedy for a variety of ailments and believed
in the results. Yet, in scientific terms, the association of the
benefits of tea drinking with tea polyphenols is rather new.
Decades ago, components such as caffeine or vitamin C were
considered the principal constituents in green tea that exert
beneficial effects on human health. In 1979, the late Dr. Isu-
neo Kada of the National Institute of Genetics in Japan found
that, among hundreds of herbal or vegetable extracts, green
tea extract showed potent bioantimutagenic effects on the
spontaneous mutations of a mutator strain of *Bacillus subtilis*
NIG1125. This fact implied that the spontaneous mutations of
DNA might be inhibited by drinking green tea and accordingly
might prevent the carcinogenesis of human cells.

I lost no time in visiting Dr. Kada's laboratory to see if I
could collaborate with him in elucidating the principal component in tea that shows antimutagenic potency. One of the routine jobs in our laboratory at that time was to analyze tea components for quality control of the products produced by our tea
blending/packaging factory. In collaboration with Dr. Kada,
we were able to elucidate the bioantimutagenic constituent in
green tea: epigallocatechin gallate, or EGCg. The high-performance liquid chromatography (HPLC) analyzer was still rare
in those days, and we had to conduct the separation of chemical components by paper chromatography. In order to confirm
the anticarcinogenic potency in vivo, we needed a good amount
of catechins, as well as laboratory animals. In those days, tea
catechin samples were not available commercially since there
was little motivation for scientists in the field of tea to study
tea catechins (pungency in green tea has been and still is regarded as something that depreciates the market price of tea).

In a corner of a factory we built a solvent separation system to derive crude catechin powder from green tea, bought a very valuable preparative HPLC system, and set up a room for rodents in a laboratory. With these facilities, I was firmly determined that we would do every possible experiment in order to prove the theory that catechins are responsible for the health benefits of tea. I had also been sending samples of pure catechins to various laboratories worldwide. To my surprise, as we conducted more experiments with tea catechins, additional new and favorable functions were discovered. We are now aware that from the basic properties of tea catechins (antioxidative, radical scavenging, protein binding, and metal chelating actions), a multitude of functions arise that battle against the deterioration of human health, particularly age-related or life-style-related malignancies.

In the sphere of cancer chemoprevention, we have made tremendous progress over recent years. Since 1996, we have been collaborating with the Department of Chemoprevention at the National Cancer Institute, National Institutes of Health, with the purpose of substantiating the green tea catechin extract (Polyphenon E) as a pharmaceutical chemopreventive agent. Although a single molecule is preferred for use as a pharmaceutical agent, the cost of producing EGCg in such a pure form is exorbitantly high. Thus, in order to prove that Polyphenon E is just as effective as pure EGCg, and to disprove the possible efficacy of the residual component in this polyphenol mixture, Phase I trials were conducted with both of these agents. Now, Chemistry, Manufacture, and Control (CMC) of Polyphenon E have been established under cGMP according to U.S. Food and Drug Administration criteria, and we are in the process of conducting Phase II trials on various types of precancerous lesion with Polyphenon E to assess its effectiveness on regression of the disorders. In years to come, we hope to be able to announce that Polyphenon E ointment or capsules are approved as a chemopreventive agent for various precancerous lesions.

The following chapters are primarily the results of the studies conducted over the past 20 years in our laboratory, as well as in our collaborative laboratories. Other relevant topics, including the historical and industrial background of tea in Japan and the research and development of the catechin industry, are also dealt with in this book.

Yukihiko Hara

Acknowledgments

Twenty years ago, in 1979, when I was working with Dr. T. Kada of the National Institute of Genetics in the search for the principal compound that showed bioantimutagenicity in green tea, no actual tea catechin samples were available anywhere, although their chemical structures were known and documented. In those days, polyphenolic compounds in tea were quantified as total polyphenols (total catechins) by the ferro-tartaric method, and no analysis was made for individual catechins. By fractionating tea brew, Ms. T. Suzuki, my assistant in those days, and I came to the conclusion that the principal antimutagenic compound was contained in the polyphenolic (catechin) fraction. As we were in need of catechin samples to determine which individual catechins were active, we visited the National Tea Research Institute. Dr. T. Takeo of the Institute was cooperative enough to discuss our situation with one of his colleagues, Mr. F. Okada, who generously provided us with several milligrams of catechins that had been earmarked for his own experiments. With these compounds, not only were Dr. Kada and I able to confirm that the individual catechin EGCg exerts bioantimutagenic action on bacterial DNA, but we were also able to develop a large-scale purification system for tea catechins. This was the beginning of my career in the study of physiological actions of tea catechins, and my work in this field continues to this day. I do recollect the names mentioned above with deep thanks.

In my position as director of the Food Research Laboratories of Mitsui Norin Co., Ltd., I have overseen the ongoing research into the physiological actions of tea. Today, about 20 full-fledged researchers with diverse expertise are working on different facets of tea research along with about 10 assistants. Over the past 20 years, there has been a constant flow of research staff who have contributed to our studies. Without the devotion of both those in the past and those who are still working in our laboratory, our work could not have reached its present stage. I sincerely express my gratitude for the devotion and endeavor of those people: S. Matsuzaki, M. Ohya, K. Okushio, H. Ishikawa, M. Watanabe, F. Tono-oka, T. Ishigami, A. Ishigaki, M. Honda, N. Matsumoto, R. Seto, F. Nanjo, and many others. At the same time, I wish to thank the many collaborators outside our laboratory, researchers in national institutes and professors at universities who expanded our realm of research. Without their guidance, our research would not have covered such a vast scope. Since so many people are involved in these extensive studies into tea polyphenols, I could not possibly mention all of these admirable people to whom I am so much indebted. Lastly, I would like to thank Ms. Andrea Kay Suzuki for her contribution in correcting the English in the manuscript.

Contents

Green Tea

1

Introduction to the History of Tea

I. ORIGINS AND BEGINNINGS

Today the tea bush is known as *Camellia sinensis* (L.) O. Kuntze of which there are two varieties: var. *sinensis* and var. *assamica*. In 1690, E. Kaempfer, a German medical doctor cum botanist who came to Japan from Holland and observed the habit of tea drinking among the people, named the bush "thea." In 1753, the famed botanist C. Linné gave to it the name of *Camellia sinensis* changing his original naming of *Thea sinensis*. Since then the nomenclature of the tea bush has been confused between these two names. In 1958, a British botanist J. R. Sealy classified all plants in the genus *Camellia* and tea was given the name it has today (1).

Tracing the origin of the tea bush is laborious work, since it spans countless numbers of geological years from the Tertiary period on and covers vast mountainous areas in southeastern Asia. General consensus attributes the birth of the tea

bush to the area we now call Southwestern China. Tea is cultivated successfully in many different countries of the world and
consumed in almost every part of the world, but for most people the association of tea with China remains strong. The discovery of a tea bush deep in Assam, India, with leaves much
larger than the Chinese one, stirred up controversy over the
original birthplace of *C. sinensis*. This discovery was made in
1823 by R. Bruce, and the bush in Assam was in later years
classified as *C. sinensis* var. *assamica*. Despite wide morphological differences between the varieties *sinensis* and *assamica* and their hybrids, genetic differences between these varieties are negligible. Today the birthplace of the tea bush is
assumed to be the Southwestern China, centered in the Yun-
nan district (2).

The history of tea drinking is another matter of controversy. Tea leaves have probably been utilized, drunk, eaten,
pickled, etc., by mountain tribes since time immemorial. The
custom's spread and acceptance among Chinese culture and
its documentation within Chinese writings are two different
matters. In other words, we have two possible approaches in
tracing the history of tea usage: anthropological or archival.
Chinese legend claims that tea consumption goes back as far
as 2737 B.C. Around that time, Sheng Nung, a legendary Em-
peror known as the Divine Healer, discovered the healing
power in tea leaves and taught people ways in which tea could
be consumed. The first credible documentary reference on tea
was made in 59 B.C. in a servant's contract, which stated that
his duties included the making of tea and going to the city to
buy it. Although it seems to be impossible to exactly pinpoint
the advent of tea drinking, the most reliable overall book on
tea was published in A.D. 780. Written by Lu Yu, who described
the botany, cultivation, and processing of tea, as well as the
utensils and proper way of drinking tea, etc., in detail, *Tea
Classics* or *Tea Sutra* and has been the Bible for people involved with tea ever since. The only contemporary counterpart
with such an encyclopedic description was published in 1935,
All About Tea, by W. Ukers (3).

II. TEA AS A PANACEA

The tea that today is commonly consumed in countries all over the world was once revered for its curative powers. Some of the earliest mentions of tea in Chinese literature refer to it as a remedy for a diverse range of complaints (4). Gradually though, tea became more and more commonly consumed and its role in society started to shift from that of a highly esteemed panacea to one of being simply a refreshing and habitual beverage.

The importance of tea for Tibetans or for nomadic people in peripheral China is something special even today. These people seem to consume much of their vital elements from tea as well as from the milk of their herd. The habit of tea drinking is so deeply ingrained in their daily life that tea has become something beyond just a beverage; they seem to have an element of addiction to tea, which is an integral part of their lives. The beneficial influence of tea on health has been felt by people since those beginning days in tea's history when it was regarded as being a cure for almost everything. Some of those claims to tea's efficacy still sound rather exaggerated, but others are, in fact, proving to have some scientific basis.

Debate on its blessings and evils has accompanied tea from the very beginning and throughout its establishment in various countries; still today there remains some controversy due to the presence of caffeine in this widely consumed beverage. China's reverence of tea was adopted by some in the Western world, but met with skepticism and outright opposition by others. The controversy was already raging in Europe in the years when tea was introduced. For as many who praised tea for its desirable effects on the body, there appeared to be as many who denounced it as being positively harmful or, at least, inconsequential.

In England during the seventeenth century, tea became famous through its introduction in the coffee shops where it was positively portrayed as a drink for good health. Advertisements in these establishments proclaimed tea's benefits to their customers. The first of these papers appeared in a coffee house (named "Garraways") run by Thomas Garway, who pioneered the sale of prepared tea in England. Among other things, it was claimed that tea was good for curing headaches, colds, fevers, and stomach problems, as well as preventing sleepiness and stimulating the appetite and digestion (3). With this persuasive advertising it is no wonder that drinking tea became such a popular pastime.

III.   TEA AS A TAXABLE PRODUCT

It is fitting that China, the country where tea was first popularized, introduced the first tea tax. This was in the eighth century under the Tang dynasty. In those years of the Tang dynasty, silk produced in China was bartered for horses bred by western nomadic tribes (5). In the following Sung dynasty, tea replaced silk, and the tea–horse barter system was established. In the Ming dynasty, this practice became so popular that in 1398 it was reported that 250 tons of tea were bartered for 13,584 horses. This shows that the production of tea was widespread in China during this time and that tea constituted a considerable revenue for the government.

In England, too, where there is no production of tea, it was the widespread use of tea that prompted the government to impose a tax. The proprietors of coffee houses were required to obtain a license and pay a duty every month. In spite of the tax, tea prospered and in time outstripped both coffee and cocoa in popularity. This seems to have been due to a number of factors, one of which was the Queen of England's partiality to tea. Catherine of Braganza, a Portuguese princess who married Charles II in 1662, brought to the English court her love of tea. Ladies of the upper class began to follow this tea-drinking fancy, which eventually spread to include members of all classes and both sexes. Another reason for tea's success could have been that the production of coffee was dominated by the Dutch, thus making it difficult for England to procure sufficient amounts. Instead, she turned her attention to establishing strong trading links in tea with Asia—and so England became a country where tea drinking was prevalent.

The United States, too, could have been a nation of tea drinkers. It started out along that track, but events of history took over to determine the destiny of tea in America. Introduced to the colonies around the middle of the seventeenth century, most probably by Dutch immigrants, tea soon produced its own fashionable culture. Tea gardens, where entertainment was provided from morning to night, came into being. All this enthusiasm was squashed, however, with the imposition of a tea tax. While it was not a large amount, rather than pay the duty, the colonists smuggled in tea from Holland. But loathe to miss out on the market in America, England put into action a more ominous plan, which allowed the British East India Company a monopoly to export tea directly from China, cutting out the middlemen. England's twofold policy of imposing a tax on one hand and monopolizing the market with cheaper teas on the other, kindled the protests of colonists, particularly those who earned their living by smuggling. For the early Americans, the prevailing opinion was that to yield to England's manipulation was to sacrifice independence.

In spite of this mood of opposition, England stubbornly refused to bend and the tea was shipped. The climax of this volatile situation in 1773 was what is now known in history as the Boston Tea Party. While the ships lay stranded in Boston harbor, forbidden to unload their cargo of tea and refused custom's clearance to sail back home, the citizens of Boston took matters into their own hands. A group of men disguised as Mohawk Indians rushed onto the ships, seized the tea chests, then proceeded to ax open each one and empty them into the sea. So it was that a menial tax marked the beginning of America's struggle for independence and was responsible for the demise of tea in America. Even today, we regard the United States as a nation of coffee drinkers, although tea has started to make a comeback with its growing reputation as a beverage conducive to promoting good health.

Another historically revolutionary incident in which tea

played a role was the opium war. In the late eighteenth century, imports of tea from China to England were steadily increasing. The British government taxed it heavily in an attempt to finance expenditures for the war in America. To curtail smuggling that arose because of the heavy tax, the tax was reduced, which in turn increased consumption. Eventually the East India Company had no silver to pay for the tea. With no better option available, they allowed opium to be cultivated in India and, in effect, bartered it for tea. This malpractice continued into the nineteenth century, and trade was expanded even more at the sacrifice of the many Chinese addicted to opium. After many vain appeals and controls attempting to ban this trade, the Ching dynasty finally arrested the addicts and confiscated the opium. The British government's retaliation for these actions by the Chinese was the opium war, which ended with the Nanching Treaty in 1842. Heavy compensation and the opening of five free ports as well as the cession of Hong Kong was the price paid by the subdued Ching dynasty. Greed for tea sacrificed many people and kept Hong Kong under foreign sovereignty for more than 100 years.

IV. DEVELOPMENT OF TEA CULTURE IN JAPAN

Tea drinking, which may have started as the preparation of a beverage from the raw leaves of wild tea trees in boiling water by mountain tribes in southern China, developed into a social rite of exquisite refinement in many parts of the world and reached its ultimate form in Japan. Early visitors from Europe in the sixteenth century found tea in China to be a popular medicinal drink, whereas in Japan they found that tea held a completely different status. They were impressed by the way people drank tea in a certain aesthetic–religious ritual. From early Japanese history, Japan has been heavily influenced by Chinese culture. Tea was introduced, along with Buddhism, from China in the eighth century or earlier. Tea growing and the habit of drinking tea then lapsed for another

400 years. A resurgence occurred, however, in the twelfth to thirteenth centuries when Buddhist priests who had studied in China brought back tea seeds and planted them in many parts of the country. Yeisai, the founder of the Rinzai sect of Zen Buddhism in Japan, wrote the first book on tea, *Tea and Health Promotion*, in 1214, in which he emphasized the virtue of tea drinking based on the experience and the beliefs he had learned in China. The Buddhist priests not only found the beverage useful for keeping them awake during their meditation, but also found that it relieved them of their physical fatigue. Tea drinking gradually spread from being popular not only among the priests and religious orders but also among the common people.

In the fifteenth to sixteenth centuries, with the advent of noted tea masters with Zen-sect Buddhist backgrounds, tea was elevated to a religion of aestheticism, teaism. Teaism is a cult founded on the worship of the beautiful, the love of nature through simplicity of materials. It is performed as "Cha-no-yu" or the tea ceremony. Tea masters such as Sen-no Rikyu in the sixteenth century, along with his predecessors and successors, perfected the art of the tea ceremony under the patronage of the then reigning lord of warring Japan. The followers of Sen-no Rikyu and other tea masters established separate schools of teaism that, even until the present day, abide by a certain decorum in the serving and appreciation of tea. Tea ceremony used to be the art of men, but today many people, particularly young women about to enter into marriage, take tea ceremony lessons and learn how to appreciate and behave in their daily life through serving tea. In the formal tea ceremony, the guests are ushered into a small and seemingly humble cottage designed to accommodate no more than five persons. A host, the tea master, who is considered to be a master of artistic life, makes and serves tea to the guests, who should appreciate the whole setting: the garden, the path, the tea house itself, the hanging scroll, the arranged flowers, the sweet cakes served, etc., as well as the tea utensils used. The tea served in the tea ceremony is called *matcha* (pronounced "mahcha") and is powdered tea of the highest quality. Matcha is beaten with lukewarm water with a whisk in a small porcelain bowl and served. It is said that teaism represents much of the art and spiritual background of Japanese life.

V. THE CHEMICAL HISTORY OF TEA

While the history of tea drinking is ancient, investigation into the chemical components of tea is in comparison quite recent. Tea is composed of unique constituents among other plants. Caffeine is found only in a few other plants other than tea. Theanine, which is unique to tea, is a kind of amino acid constituting more than half the total amount of amino acids in tea. Major catechins in tea are also unique to tea. Vitamin C was found to be contained in tea after it was discovered in lemons. Tea aroma is an area that attracted the interest of scientists who had been seeking one single compound that represents tea, a search which has yet been in vain. In 1827 caffeine was discovered in tea. At that time it was given the name theine, but when it was proven that the structure and properties of this substance were exactly the same as caffeine that was identified in coffee in 1820, the name theine was dropped. In 1924, vitamin C was discovered in green tea by two Japanese scientists, M. Miura and M. Tsujimura, under Professor U. Suzuki.

The astringency of tea, too, was investigated extensively by Tsujimura. In the years 1927 to 1935, Tsujimura isolated epicatechin, epicatechin gallate, and epigallocatechin. With great effort, she purified them and determined their structural formulas. In 1950, with the new technique of column chromatography, the British scientist A. B. Bradfield succeeded in isolating epigallocatechin gallate and determined its structure by x-ray diffraction method. Tsujimura later identified her compound as being the same. Thus, the main four catechins in tea, which make up the major group of compounds in the soluble solids of tea, were identified in the early 1950s and Tsujimura, along with Bradfield, gained worldwide renown for their pioneering work. Later in the 1950s, E. A. H. Roberts clarified the steric complications of individual catechins in Britain, using the technique of two-dimensional paper chromatography. He is also known for his research on polyphenolic compounds, theaflavins, and thearubigins in black tea. Later, around 1963–1965, Y. Takino et al. confirmed the benzotropolone structure of theaflavins. The chemistry of tea polyphenols in that of broader plant polyphenols was well reviewed by E. Haslam (6).

Aroma components in tea were first researched more than 150 years ago by Mulder, who discovered essential oil in fresh tea leaves. In the 1930s, S. Takei and R. Yamamoto et al. were among the earliest scientists to contribute to our knowledge of tea aroma. Methods at that time were rather crude and tons of tea, not to mention time and patience, were necessary to isolate sufficient material for separation and identification of individual components. The work of these professors (Takei, who focused mainly on green tea, and Yamamoto, who focused on Taiwan black tea) became a vital basis for future research in the field. They identified more than 30 compounds from green and black teas. Following in their steps, T. Yamanishi, successor of Professor Tsujimura, also became renowned worldwide for her work, which involved isolating aroma components by gas chromatography (5). Today more than 600 aroma compounds have been identified.

Theanine, γ-ethylamide of glutamic acid, was discovered in 1950 by Y. Sakato. Theanine constitutes the "umami" or sweet taste in tea, particularly that of Gyokuro (the best quality green tea in Japan, see Chapter 20), and constitutes 2% of tea. The antagonistic action of theanine against the stimulating action of caffeine in the nervous system and its vitalizing action on brain neurons are areas of interest that could be studied further.

REFERENCES

1. JR Sealy. A Revision of the Genus *Camellia*. London: The Royal Horticultural Society, 1958.
2. S Yamaguchi, JI Tanaka. Origin and Spread of Tea from China

to Eastern Asian Regions and Japan. Proceeding of '95 International Tea-Quality-Human Health Symposium, Shanghai, China, Nov. 7–10, 1995, pp 279–286.

3. WH Ukers. All About Tea. New York: The Tea and Coffee Trade Journal Company, 1935.
4. L Hu. Medicinal Tea and Medicinal Syrup. Beijing: Traditional Chinese Medicine Ancient Books Press, 1986, pp 1–2.
5. T Yamanishi. Special issue on tea. Food Reviews International, 11:3, 1995.
6. E Haslam. Plant Polyphenols, Vegetable Tannins Revisited. Cambridge: Cambridge University Press, 1989.

2

Biosynthesis of Tea Catechins

The tea plant contains many kinds of polyphenols, catechins being particularly prolific. Catechins belong to those groups of compounds generically known as flavonoids, which have a C_6-C_3-C_6 carbon structure and are composed of two aromatic rings, A and B (Fig. 1). Currently, the tea plant is known to contain seven kinds of major catechins and traces of various other catechin derivatives. They are divided into two classes: the free catechins, (+)-catechin, (+)-gallocatechin, (−)-epicatechin, (−)-epigallocatechin; and the esterified or galloyl catechins, (−)-epicatechin gallate, (−)-epigallocatechin gallate, (−)-gallocatechin gallate, (Fig. 2). While the galloyl catechins are astringent (EGCg, ECg) with a bitter aftertaste (ECg), free catechins have far less astringency (EGC, EC), leaving a slightly sweet aftertaste (EGC) even at 0.1% aqueous solutions.

These catechins are present in all parts of the tea plant; 15–30% are present in the tea shoots, and there is also a high content in the second and third leaves. In August, when the sun's rays are the strongest, catechin content is the highest.

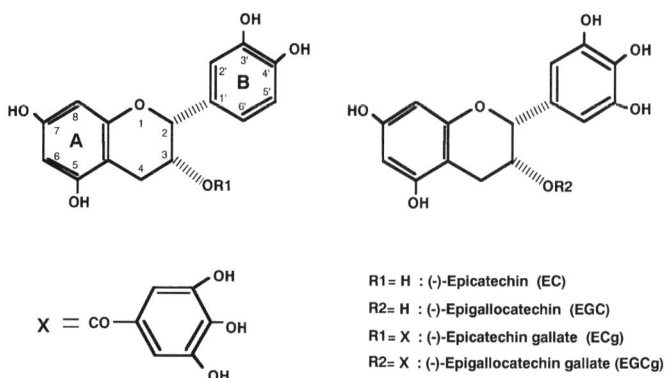

FIG. 1   The basic structural formulas of tea catechins.

Synthesis of tea catechins was researched by Zaprometov (1). When $^{14}CO_2$ is assimilated with the tea leaves for 2 hours, ^{14}C could be traced in the four main catechins. As time passes, the formation of free catechins decreases and the galloyl catechins increase. Catechin formation is prolific in the bud and upper leaves.

Biosynthesis of catechins is shown in Fig. 3. The C_6 (A) catechin ring is produced by the acetic–malonic acid pathway and C_3-C_6 (B) is produced by the shikimic–cinnamic acid pathway starting from the glucose pool. This fact was discovered during research into the synthesis of rutin (quercetin) in soba (buckwheat flour). When ^{14}C-acetic acid is supplied, metabolism occurs only at the A-ring of quercetin, and when ^{14}C-shikimic acid or ^{14}C-t-cinnamic acid is supplied, ^{14}C occurs at the C_3-C_6 structure. In this way the C_6-C_3-C_6 structure of flavanoid is synthesized with the decarboxylation of three molecules of acetic-malonyl-CoA and cinnamic-coumaroyl-CoA. The first stable C_6-C_3-C_6 compound is confirmed to be chalcone from which catechin is synthesized by way of flavanone.

(−)-Epigallocatechin is produced by hydroxylation of (−)-epicatechin. Then (−)-epicatechin gallate and (−)-epigallocatechin gallate are synthesized by esterification of catechins with gallic acid (2).

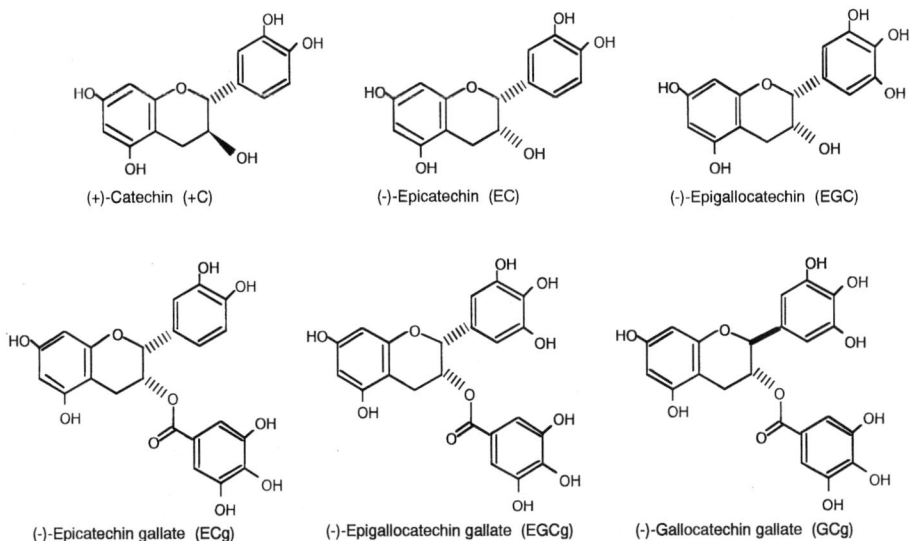

(+)-Catechin (+C)   (-)-Epicatechin (EC)   (-)-Epigallocatechin (EGC)

(-)-Epicatechin gallate (ECg)   (-)-Epigallocatechin gallate (EGCg)   (-)-Gallocatechin gallate (GCg)

FIG. 2   The structural formulas of catechins.

It was confirmed that carbons in the N-ethyl group of theanine are incorporated into catechin (3), although this pathway of catechin synthesis seems to be a minor one.

The catechin content of the tea plant varies according to the variety of the plant. In black tea varieties the catechin content makes up 30% of the dried matter and in green tea varieties it is up to 20%. In both varieties there are also differences in the activities of enzymes involved in biosynthesis.

The production of catechins in the tea plant increases on exposure to light and decreases in the shade. These phenomena are related to the activity of phenylalanine-ammonia-lyase, which is a key enzyme in the biosynthesis of catechin B ring. When the tea plant is covered (blocking out light), this enzyme activity decreases rapidly.

The biosynthesis of catechin is also increased by a rise in temperature. Once catechin is synthesized, it is stored in the vacuole of the cell and hardly undergoes any metabolism or decomposition.

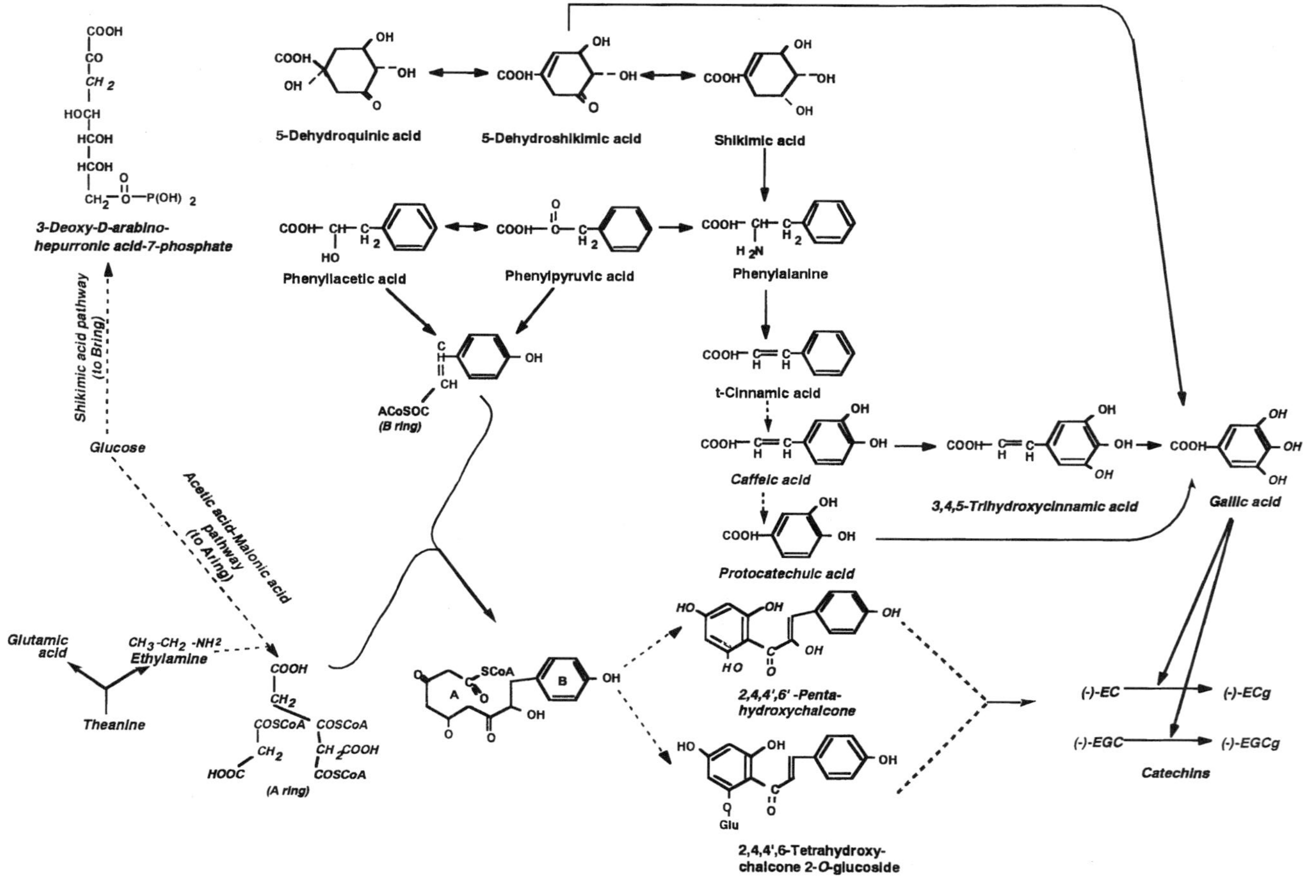

FIG. 3 The biosynthetic pathway of catechins in tea leaves.

REFERENCES

1. MN Zaprometov, AL Kursanov. Figiologia Rastenii 5:51–61, 1958.
2. K Iwasa. Biosynthesis of catechins in tea plant. Bulletin of the National Res Inst of Tea 13:101–126, 1977.
3. M Kito, H Kokura, J Izaki, K Sasaoka. Theanine, a precursor of the phloroglucinol nucleus of catechins in tea plants. Phytochem 7:599–603, 1968.

3

Fermentation of Tea

Black tea is manufactured according to the process shown in Fig. 1. First, the freshly plucked leaves are withered overnight in the trough to reduce their moisture content to almost half. Withering is an important process in producing the fragrance of tea, and it renders the leaves more pliable for rolling, the next process. During the rolling process, polyphenol oxidase (PO) and catechins, which exist separately in the tea leaf, mix. The polyphenols (catechins) are located in vacuole in the palisade layer of the tea leaves, whereas the enzyme is located in the epidermal layer. During the process of fermentation, enzymatic oxidation occurs with catechins forming dimers or highly complexed groups of compounds. These oxidized products represent the reddish-brown colors of black tea.

In 1957, E. A. H. Roberts revealed two-dimensional paper chromatograms with two orange-colored spots and one reddish-brown tailing spot. He termed the former and its

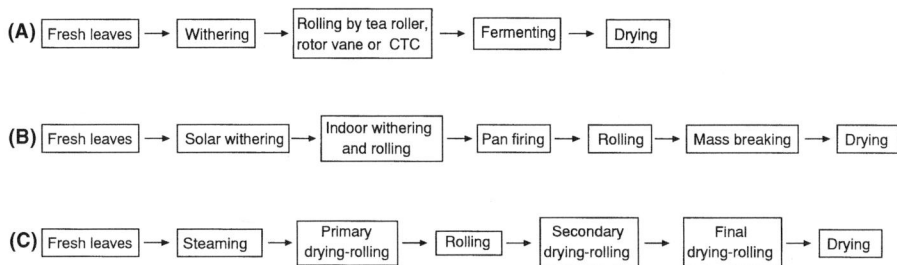

FIG. 1 The manufacturing processes of tea: (A) black tea; (B) oolong tea; and (C) green tea (Sen-cha).

gallate "theaflavin" and the latter "thearubigin" (1). He developed a method in which individual catechins (precursors) were mixed with polyphenol oxidase and the resultant spots on the paper chromatograph were compared with those obtained from the infusion of black tea. In this way, he postulated the existence of bisflavanols in addition to theaflavins. In theaflavins, he confirmed the existence of benzotropolone structure. Thus, Roberts' research was pioneering in that it triggered subsequent research on the chemical reactions of black tea (2).

In 1963, Y. Takino et al. obtained crystals by reacting (−)-EC and (−)-EGCg in the presence of polyphenol oxidase (3). He confirmed the crystal to be the same compound as Roberts' theaflavin. He postulated the formation pathway of theaflavins from catechins as shown in Fig. 2. Polyphenol oxidase takes part only in the initial formation of quinones and reactions thereafter proceed automatically. Fig. 3 shows the main four kinds of theaflavins that in total make up 1–2% of black tea on a dry-weight basis.

Thearubigin is formed by the polymerization of catechins and makes up 10–20% of black tea which is 10 to 20 times greater than the dry weight of the theaflavins. The chemical structure of thearubigin is still unknown. It is a heterogeneous group of compounds with a molecular weight of 700–40,000.

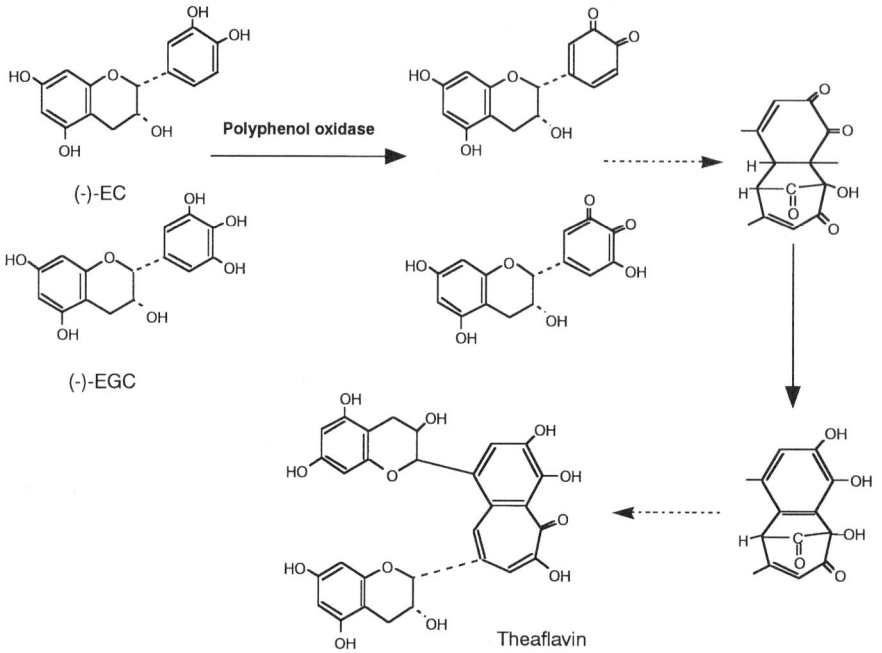

FIG. 2 Proposed biosynthesis of theaflavins.

It is confirmed that thearubigins have no benzotropolone ring, as opposed to theaflavins. The degradation of thearubigin fraction renders flavan-3-ols, flavan-3-ol gallates, antocyanidin, delphinidin and gallic acid, as well as polysaccharide and protein residues (4). This action suggests that in the process of fermentation, catechins, proanthocyanidins and degraded theaflavins might form a dialysable low molecule thearubigin at first, and then further polymerization and complexation with protein or polysaccharide occur to form undialysable thearubigin. It is said that the higher the content of theaflavins, the better price the tea fetches. This is not always true. Many other factors also contribute to determining the market price of black tea, although a high theaflavin content usually implies good manufacturing practices.

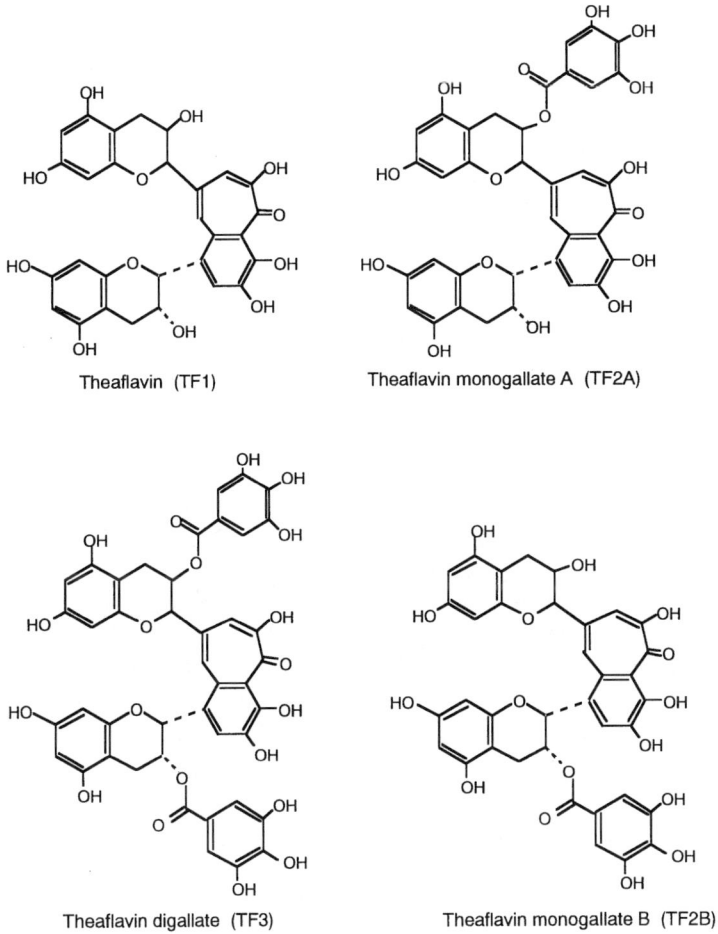

FIG. 3   Structural formulas of theaflavins.

Oolong tea, which is partly fermented, contains a lesser
amount of catechins than green tea and a lesser amount of
theaflavins than black tea. Oolong tea, as well as black tea,
have characteristic bisflavanols, i.e., theasinensins. As shown
in Fig. 4, Nishioka et al. identified three kinds of theasinensins in black tea (A, B, C), and four additional kinds in oolong

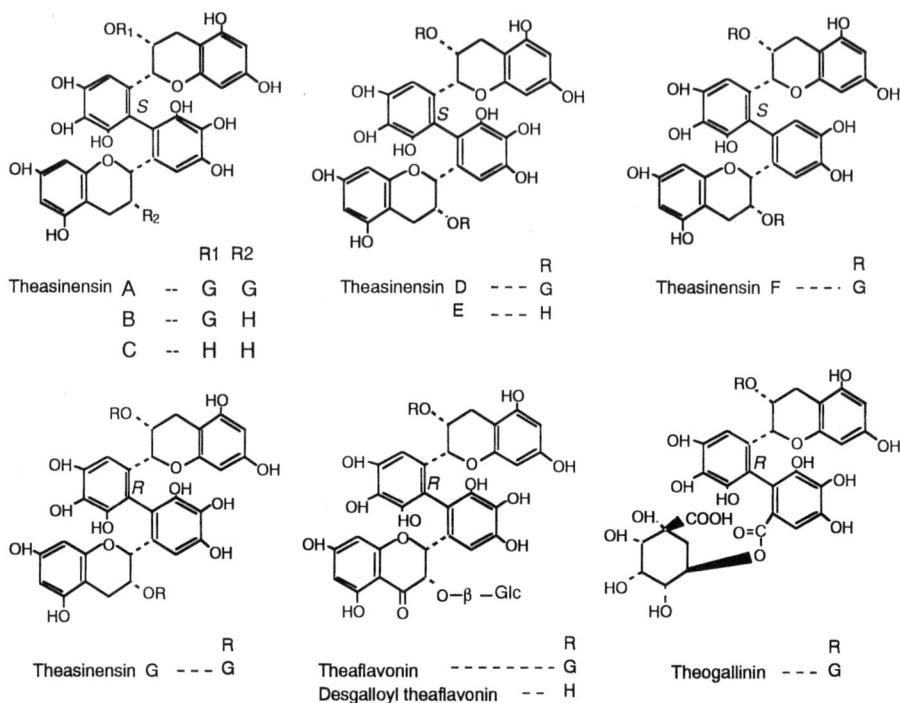

FIG. 4   Structural formulas of theasinensis.

tea (D, E, F, G), as well as theaflavonins and theogallinin in black tea (5).

REFERENCES

1. EAH Roberts, RA Cartwright, M Oldschool. The Phenolic Substances of Manufactured Tea. J Sci Food Agric 8:72–80, 1957.
2. EAH Roberts. Economic importance of flavonoid substances: tea fermentation. In: TA Geissman, ed. The Chemistry of Flavonoid Compounds. New York: The Macmillan Company, 1962, pp 468–512.
3. Y Takino, H Imagawa. Studies on the oxidation of catechins by tea oxidase formation of a crystalline reddish orange pigment of benzotropolone nature. Agr Biol Chem 27:319–321, 1963.

4. T Ozawa, M Kataoka, O Negishi. Elucidation of the partial structure of polymeric thearubigins from black tea. Biosci Biotechnol Biochem 60:2023–2027, 1996.
5. G Nonaka, O Kawahara, I Nishioka. Tannins and related compounds. XV. A New Class of Dimeric Flavan-3-ol Gallates, Theasinensins A and B, and Proanthocyanidin Gallates from Green Tea Leaf. (1). Chem Pharm Bull 31:3906–3914, 1983.

4

Methods of Extracting Polyphenolic Constituents of Tea Leaves

I. CATECHINS

In green tea, the polyphenolic fraction is mostly composed of catechins; they are the major components of fresh tea leaves, as well as of the soluble matter in green tea. Crude catechin powder is obtainable by treating tea leaves with water and organic solvents, as shown in Fig. 1. The total catechin content of this crude product is a little more than 90%. The green tea catechin (GTC) fraction is then submitted to liquid chromatography to isolate four different catechin compounds (1). The composition of the GTC fraction is shown in Table 1.

The production of tea catechin fractions may be accomplished, however, without the use of any harmful solvents. Such methods are presently employed to produce green tea extracts of various grades for commercial purposes under the trademark of Polyphenon™. All future references to GTC in this book are referring to Polyphenon 100™ (with more than 90% catechin purity and caffeine-free). In commercial produc-

Green tea
     Extracted with hot water
     Spray dried

Water-soluble green tea powder
     Dissolved in hot water
     Washed with chloroform

Aqueous layer   Chloroform layer
     Extracted with ethyl acetate

Ethyl acetate layer   Aqueous layer
     Evaporated

Conc. solution
     Freeze dried

Green tea catechin

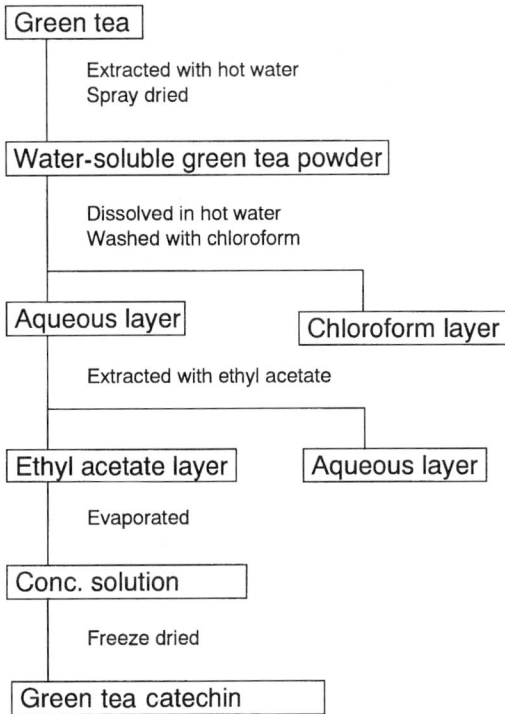

FIG. 1 The preparation of green tea catechins.

TABLE 1 Composition of Green Tea Catechins

Catechins	Absolute (%)	Relative (%)
(+)-Gallocatechin (+GC)	1.4	1.6
(−)-Epigallocatechin (EGC)	17.57	19.3
(−)-Epicatechin (EG)	5.81	6.4
(−)-Epigallocatechin gallate (EGCg)	53.90	59.1
(−)-Epicatechin gallate (ECg)	12.51	13.7
Total	91.23	100

Black tea

    Extracted with hot water
    Spray dried

Water-soluble black tea powder

    Dissolved in hot water
    Washed with chloroform

Aqueous layer   Chloroform layer

    Extracted with methyl *iso*-butyl ketone (M*i* Bk)

M*i* BK layer   Aqueous layer

    Evaporated

Conc. solution

    Freeze dried

Crude theaflavins

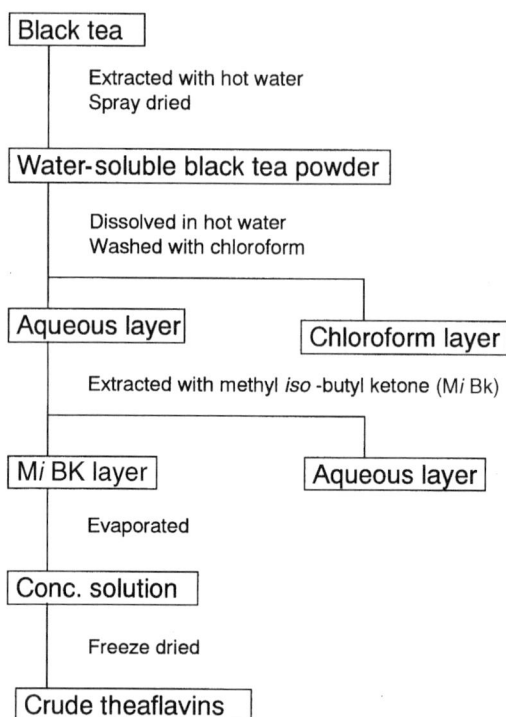

FIG. 2   The preparation of crude theaflavins.

TABLE 2   Composition of Crude Theaflavins

Theaflavins	Absolute (%)	Relative (%)
Theaflavin (TF1)	13.35	15.8
Theaflavin monogallate A (TF2A)	18.92	22.4
Theaflavin monogallate B (TF2B)	18.64	22.0
Theaflavin digallate (TF3)	33.46	39.7
Total	84.40	100

tion, Polyphenon E™, which is spray dried under cGMP, is almost the equivalent of Polyphenon 100™.

II. THEAFLAVINS

In the process of manufacturing black tea, catechins are mostly oxidized to form such pigments as theaflavins or thearubigins. In the case of tropical black tea, these fractions exist in the ratio of 15–20% thearubigins, 1–2% theaflavins, and 5–10% catechins on a dry-weight basis. The amount of theaflavins is quoted to be closely related to the commercial value of black tea. To separate theaflavins, black tea is extracted with water, then washed with solvents to remove the impurities (2). An extraction process of crude theaflavins and the composition of individual theaflavins are shown in Fig. 2 and Table 2.

REFERENCES

1. T Matsuzaki, Y Hara. Antioxidative activity of tea leaf catechins. Nippon Nogeikagaku Kaishi 59:129–134, 1985.
2. Y Hara, T Matsuzaki, T Suzuki. Angiotensin converting enzyme inhibitory activity of tea components. Nippon Nogeikagaku Kaishi 61:803–808, 1987.

5

Antioxidative Action of Tea Polyphenols

I. INTRODUCTION

Possible applications for tea catechins in numerous fields continue to grow as more and more is discovered about their antioxidative action. Since oxidative reactions are regarded as being detrimental to the body, extensive research over recent years has been undertaken to seek out ways of combating these processes. Various different compounds found in all kinds of plants, vegetables, and fruits have been found to have antioxidative action. Among these are the polyphenols exclusive to tea, which have been proved to be even more effective than some well-known and commonly used antioxidants. Both in vitro and in vivo experiments have given positive results, broadening the possibilities for practical applications.

II. ANTIOXIDATIVE ACTION IN LARD

Oxidative reactions occur not only within our bodies but also in our food, causing deterioration of freshness and quality before consumption. Tackling this problem is an extremely important issue for the food industry. Various antioxidants have been used in the past, including both those derived from natural sources and those synthetically produced. BHA, an effective antioxidant previously used worldwide, is suspended from use in several countries now because of possible carcinogenicity, although this is almost certainly unlikely under practical conditions of use. Vitamin E, while considered as being completely safe, is more costly and its usage is limited because of its lipophilic properties.

Catechins derived from tea leaves are natural, safe for consumption, and have been proved to be very effective antioxidants. Green tea catechin (GTC) and four main individual components of GTC, $(-)$-epicatechin (EC), $(-)$-epigallocatechin (EGC), $(-)$-epicatechin gallate (ECg), and $(-)$-epigallocatechin gallate (EGCg) were examined for their antioxidativity (1,2). GTC was added to lard at concentrations of 10 ppm, 20 ppm, or 50 ppm. For comparison, dl-α-tocopherol at 200 ppm and BHA at 50 ppm were also used. The peroxide value (POV) was measured using the active oxygen method (AOM). In this method, lard in a glass cylinder is heated continuously in a silicon oil bath at a temperature of $97.8°C$ with continuous bubbling air from the deeply inserted tube. The lard used was mainly composed of oleic acid ($C_{18:1}$) 43.1%, palmitic acid ($C_{16:0}$) 23.8%, stearic acid ($C_{18:0}$) 13.9%, and linoleic acid ($C_{18:2}$) 10.0%. After an induction period of a few hours the lard becomes rancid as a result of oxidation processes. However, when catechins were introduced to this system the induction period was prolonged markedly, indicating their antioxidative action. As shown in Fig. 1, green tea catechins at just 10 ppm had the same degree of antioxidativity as dl-α-tocopherol at 200 ppm.

In the same way, the four main catechins in the following concentrations were compared with dl-α-tocopherol at 200 ppm and BHA at 50 ppm: EC–50 ppm, EGC–20 ppm, ECg–50 ppm, and EGCg–20 ppm. Again, catechins were confirmed to have strong antioxidative effects (Fig. 2). Antioxidativity was in the order of EGC > EGCg > EC > ECg > BHA > dl-α-tocopherol. On a molarity basis, antioxidativity decreased

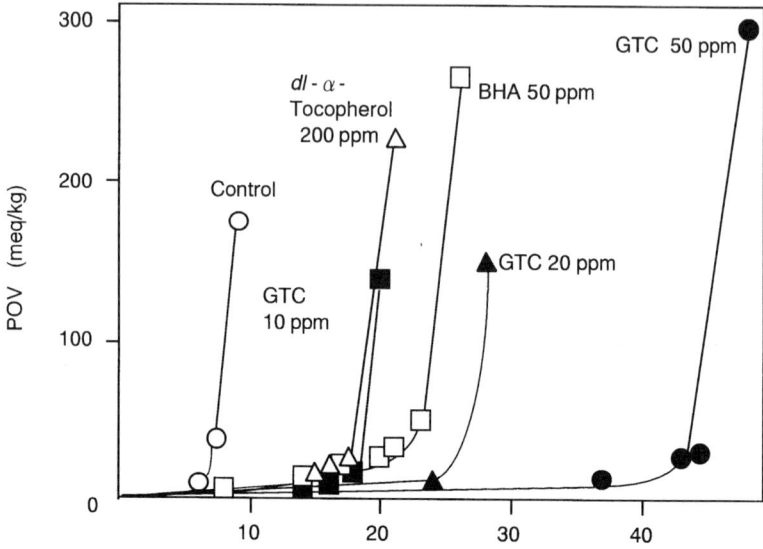

FIG. 1 Antioxidative activity of green tea catechins on lard (AOM at 97.8°C).

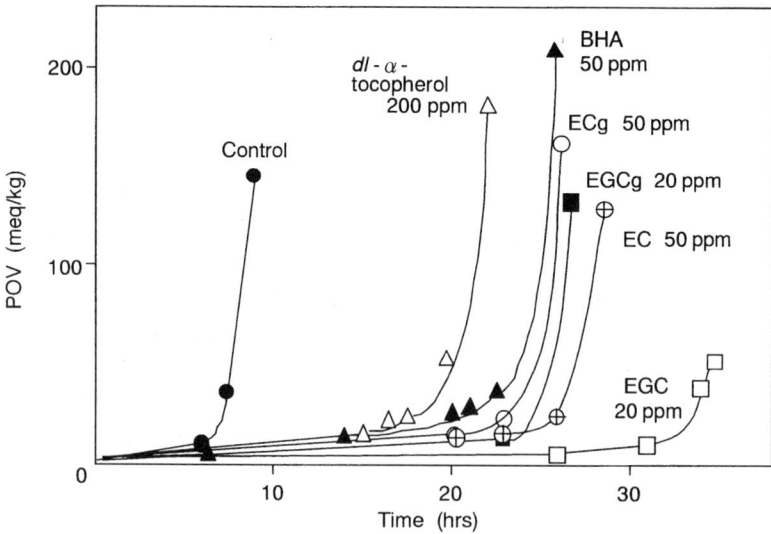

FIG. 2 Antioxidative activity of tea catechins on lard (AOM at 97.8°C).

in the following order: EGCg > EGC > ECg > EC. These results imply that the antioxidativity of catechins is related to their structure. In particular, the presence of a hydroxy group at 5' position appears to increase antioxidativity (1). Polyphenols with a pyrogallol structure, that is, with a hydroxy group at 5' position, namely EGC and EGCg, have three times the antioxidative power than polyphenols with a catechol structure such as EC and ECg, which have no hydroxy group at the 5' position.

III. SYNERGISM OF TEA CATECHINS

Synergism of EGCg with organic acids, L-ascorbic acid, tocopherol, and amino acids was investigated (3). Certain organic acids showed synergism with tea catechins. EGCg (10 ppm) was added to lard followed by the addition of 50 ppm malic acid, citric acid, and tartaric acid respectively. At AOM (97.8°C) oxidation was apparent. Twenty hours later the POV value was calculated. Results, as shown in Table 1, indicate that EGCg has a synergistic effect with all three of these organic acids.

To lard containing 5 ppm EGCg, L-ascorbic acid was added at concentrations of 5 ppm and 50 ppm respectively. Citric acid and malic acid at a concentration of 50 ppm were also observed for comparison. Results showed that the synergistic effect of EGCg with L-ascorbic acid was greater than that of EGCg with citric acid and malic acid (Table 2).

TABLE 1   Antioxidative Activity of EGCg on Lard
(Synergism with Organic Acids)

EGCg (ppm)	Organic acids (50 ppm)	POV[a] (meq/kg)
10	—	186
10	Malic acid	32
10	Citric acid	21
10	Tartaric acid	25

[a] Peroxide value (after 20 hrs by AOM at 97.8°C).

TABLE 2   Antioxidative Activity of EGCg on Lard
(Synergism with L-Ascorbic Acid)

EGCg (ppm)	Sample	(ppm)	Time[a] (days)
—	—		7.1
5	—		12.1
—	L-Ascorbic acid	50	10.9
5	L-Ascorbic acid	5	13.7
5	L-Ascorbic acid	50	16.9
5	Citric acid	50	13.8
5	Malic acid	50	14.1

[a] Number of days taken for peroxide value to reach 20 meq/kg by
AOM at 60°C).

Tocopherol was also found to have a synergistic effect
with EGCg. 100 ppm of tocopherol mix containing 60% natural
tocopherols (30% α-tocopherol and 30% other tocopherols) was
added to lard containing 5 ppm EGCg. The time taken for the
peroxide value to reach 20 meq/kg was longer than when 200
ppm tocopherol mix without EGCg was used (Table 3).

EGCg (10 ppm) was added to lard with individual amino
acids (100 ppm). Among the amino acids tested only L-methio-
nine showed slight synergism with EGCg, whereas most of the
others worked adversely.

TABLE 3   Antioxidative Activity of EGCg on Lard
(Synergism with Tocopherol Mix)

EGC (ppm)	Tocopherol mix[a] (ppm)	Time[b] (hrs)
—	—	8.0
5	—	14.8
5	100	29.0
—	200	20.0

[a] Tocopherol mix contains 60% natural tocopherol (30% α-
tocopherol and 30% others).
[b] Time taken for peroxide value to reach 20 meq/kg by AOM
at 97.8°C.

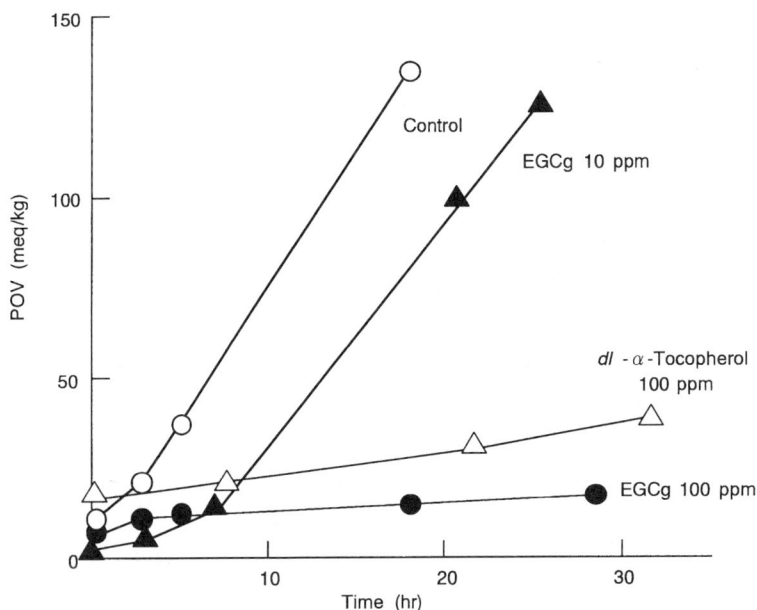

FIG. 3 Antioxidative activity of EGCg at 30°C on linoleic acid.

IV. SUPPRESSION OF PEROXIDATION OF LINOLEIC ACID

In linoleic acid EGCg also acted as an antioxidant, although its activity was not as strong as in the lard system. The antioxidative action of EGCg was confirmed, too, in a system where linoleic acid was solubilized in a large amount of water, proving its antioxidativity in both an oil and an aqueous system (Fig. 3) (1).

V. SUPPRESSION OF PHOTO-OXIDATION

An antioxidative effect against photo-oxidation by tea polyphenols was observed. Ethyl linoleate was exposed under xenon fademeter to facilitate photo-oxidation. As shown in Fig. 4, the addition of 100 ppm GTC suppressed the POV value

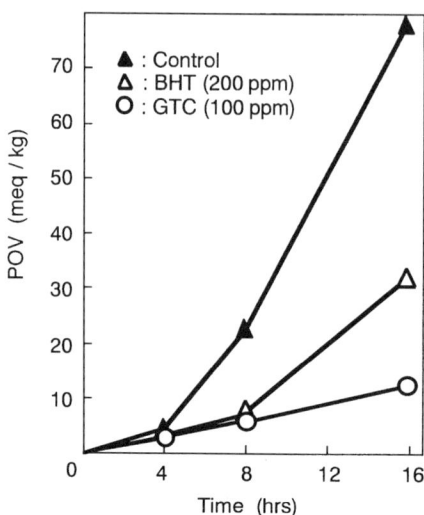

FIG. 4   Inhibition of photo-oxidation of ethyl linoleate by green tea catechins.

much more effectively than 200 ppm of BHT, a synthetic antioxidant.

VI.   INFLUENCE OF CATECHIN FEEDING ON THE LEVELS OF α-TOCOPHEROL, TBARS IN PLASMA, AND ERYTHROCYTES (4)

In order to investigate the influence of catechin feeding in a
diet rich with saturated or polyunsaturated fatty acid, male
Wistar rats 5 weeks of age were fed on the following four diets
for 31 days: 30% palm oil diet; 30% palm oil diet containing
1% GTC; 30% perilla oil diet; 30% perilla oil diet containing
1% GTC. Each group consisted of six rats and all rats were
caged individually. The composition of the diets in each group
is shown in Table 4, and the composition of fatty acids in palm
and perilla oils is shown in Table 5. To each diet, α-tocopherol
was added to give the same concentration of 6 mg/100 g, taking into account the intrinsic amount already contained in the

TABLE 4   Composition of High Fat Diets

Ingredient	Palm oil group		Perilla oil group	
	Control	GTC	Control	GTC
Corn starch (%)	28.9	28.9	28.9	28.9
Sucrose (%)	10.0	10.0	10.0	10.0
Casein (%)	20.0	20.0	20.0	20.0
Palm oil (%)	30.0	30.0	—	—
Perilla oil (%)	—	—	30.0	30.0
Cellulose (%)	5.0	5.0	5.0	5.0
Salt mixture[a] (%)	4.0	4.0	4.0	4.0
Choline chloride (%)	0.1	0.1	0.1	0.1
Vitamin mixture[a] (%)				
(Vitamin E free)	2.0	2.0	2.0	2.0
GTC (%)	—	1.0	—	1.0
α-Tocopherol[b] (mg)	3.7	3.7	4.3	4.3

[a] Salt mixture and vitamin mixture (vitamin E free) according to Harper were purchased from Oriental Kobo Kogyo Co.
[b] Taking into account the content of α-tocopherol in the palm and perilla oils, the final concentration of the α-tocopherol in the diets was adjusted to 6mg/100mg.

oils. Food and water were fed ad libitum. At the end of the feeding period, rats were fasted overnight, anesthetized, and blood was collected by heart puncture. The plasma and red blood cells were separated. During the feeding period, there were no significant differences among the groups tested in terms of either body weight gain or food intake. The effects of

TABLE 5   Fatty Acid Composition of Palm and Perilla Oils

Fatty acid	Palm oil (%)	Perilla oil (%)
14:0 Myristic	1.1	—
16:0 Palmitic	46.6	6.7
16:1 Palmitoleic	—	—
18:0 Stearic	3.8	2.1
18:1 Oleic	37.5	17.7
18:2 Linoleic	9.8	15.5
18:3 Linolenic	—	52.6
20:0 Arachidic	0.2/99.0	—/94.6

dietary tea catechins on the levels of both α-tocopherol and thiobarbituric acid-reactive substances (TBARS), an indicator of lipid peroxidation, in the plasma and erythrocytes were examined as well as the plasma lipid levels.

The plasma lipid levels in the perilla oil-fed rats were markedly lower than those in the palm oil rats, regardless of tea catechin supplementation. In perilla oil groups, significant reduction of cholesterol was noted by tea catechin supplementation (Table 6). In both of the two oil groups, TBARS content in erythrocytes was not influenced very much by catechin supplementation. However, there was a big difference between TBARS in plasma between the two oil groups as shown in Fig. 5. Perilla oil (polyunsaturated) groups, showed much higher TBARS values than those of palm oil (saturated) groups while in perilla oil groups, tea catechin supplementation suppressed TBARS significantly.

The concentration of α-tocopherol was examined in four groups and the results are shown in Fig. 6. It is apparent that the content of α-tocopherol was much lower in the perilla oil-fed group. Polyunsaturated oil (perilla oil) seems to consume more α-tocopherol than saturated oil does because of its sus-

TABLE 6 Concentration of Cholesterol, Phospholipids, and Triglycerides in Plasma

Lipids	Palm oil group		Perilla oil group	
	Control	GTC	Control	GTC
Cholesterol (mg/dl)	65.9 ± 2.7	66.7 ± 10.0	36.8 ± 2.9[a]	24.7 ± 5.0[a,b]
Phospholipids (mg/dl)	126.9 ± 11.4	121.1 ± 9.5	68.0 ± 14.9[a]	61.7 ± 11.1[a]
Triglycerides (mg/dl)	80.3 ± 10.7	67.3 ± 16.3	32.2 ± 8.0[a]	26.3 ± 3.7[a]

Values were expressed as mean ± S.D.
[a] Statistically significant differences compared with palm oil group, $p < 0.01$
[b] Statistically significant differences compared with perilla oil group, $p < 0.001$.

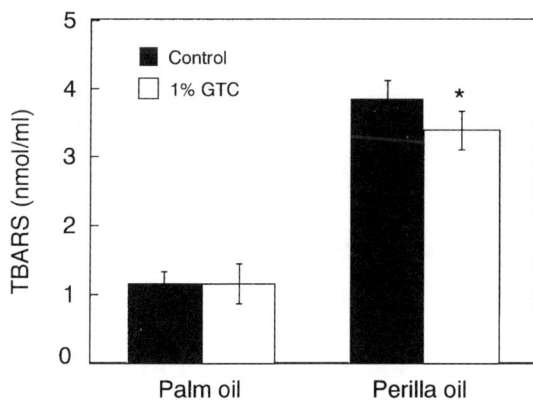

FIG. 5 Effects of green tea catechins on plasma peroxides in a 30% oil diet fed for four weeks. *Significantly different from ($p < 0.05$).

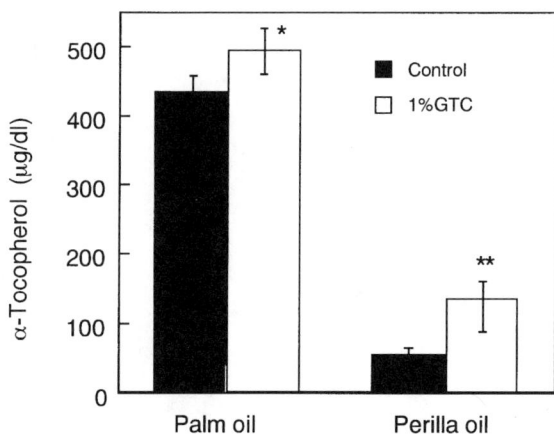

FIG. 6 Effects of green tea catechins on plasma α-tocopherol in a 30% oil diet fed for four weeks. *Significantly different from ($p < 0.05$). **Significantly different from control ($p < 0.01$).

ceptibility to oxidation. Yet the supplementation of catechins inhibits the consumption of α-tocopherol significantly in the plasma and erythrocytes. These phenomena suggest that oxidative damage in the body can be ameliorated by the supplementation of tea catechins in the diet.

VII. PRACTICAL APPLICATIONS

The strong antioxidative action of tea polyphenols opens up many opportunities for their use in a variety of practical situations, particularly in the food industry. Several examples of such commercial uses follow.

A. Antioxidative Action in Edible Oils

Green tea was added to salad oil containing about 600 ppm natural tocopherol, in concentrations of 50 ppm and 200 ppm respectively, while 200 ppm *dl*-α-tocopherol and 50 ppm BHA were used as controls. As the results in Fig. 7 show, *dl*-α-

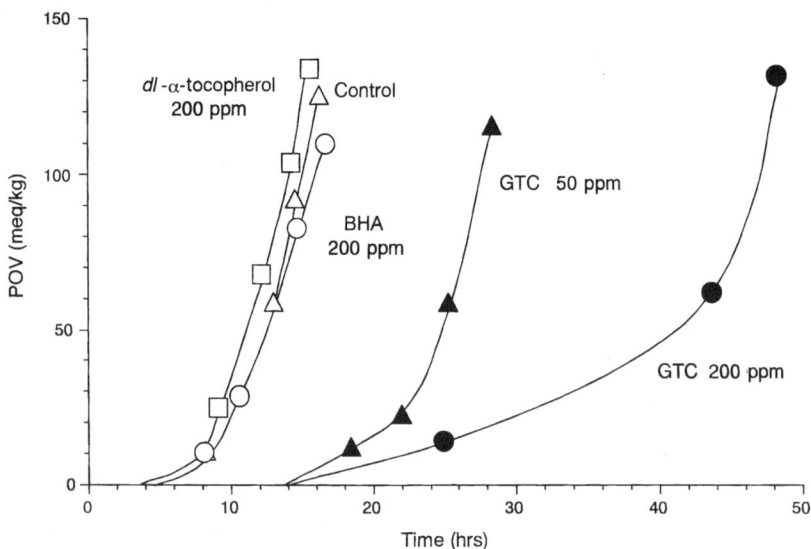

FIG. 7 Antioxidative activity of green tea catechins on salad oil (AOM at 97.8°C).

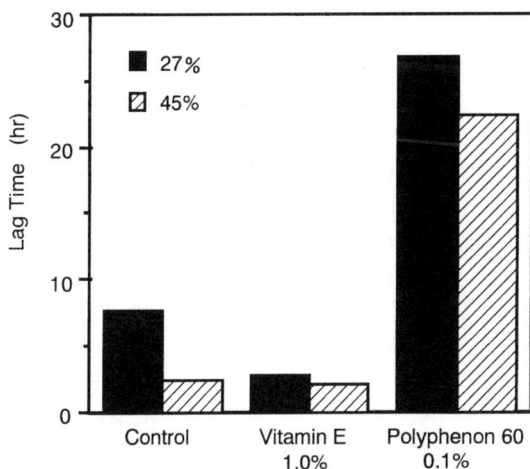

FIG. 8 Prolongation of peroxidation of fish oil containing DHA by vitamin E (27% or 45%) or tea catechins as measured by rancimat method.

tocopherol and BHA showed no antioxidativity but GTC dose-dependently inhibited the oxidation of the salad oil (5). The fact that tea catechins, unlike BHA, inhibited the oxidation of salad oil (containing tocopherol), shows there is great potential for them to be put to practical use in the food industry.

Tea catechins have been shown to be resistant to heat in fats and oils and to retain their antioxidative potency. It was also confirmed that catechins are not easily destroyed in the frying process, at 180°C for a substantial period of time. The oxidation process in fish oil containing docosahexaenoic acid (DHA) was also found to be inhibited by the 0.1% addition of tea catechins (Polyphenon 60™, a powder of more than 60% catechins) as measured by the rancimat method (Fig. 8). Thus, while vitamin E has been almost ineffective in edible oils such as soybean, rapeseed, and fish oils, tea catechins have been found to have a strong antioxidative effect.

B. Suppression of Discoloration of Natural Colors

Natural food colorings are highly valued in the food industry because of their safety and the fact that they give a truer color than chemically synthesized food colorings. However, their color stability is often inferior, which reduces their potential use. Catechins were investigated for their effectiveness in inhibiting loss of color in natural food colorings. The addition of catechins was found to be effective in the following natural food colorings (3): gardenier coloring matter, cochineal coloring matter, monascus coloring matter, natural chlorophyll, riboflavin, and β-carotene.

In a separate test with β-carotene, 10 mg was added to 100 g corn oil with 300 ppm of Polyphenon 60. The solution was put in a glass container and was kept in an ambient condition in a room. The β-carotene content in the corn oil was measured at 2-day intervals by HPLC and the amount remaining was calculated. As can be seen from Fig. 9 deterioration of β-carotene was strongly inhibited in the presence of catechins. Catechins may be added to commercially produced drinks containing β-carotene to prevent discoloration. Catechins have also been proven to be effective in retaining the fresh red color of fish such as salmon. Fish soaked overnight in a brine solu-

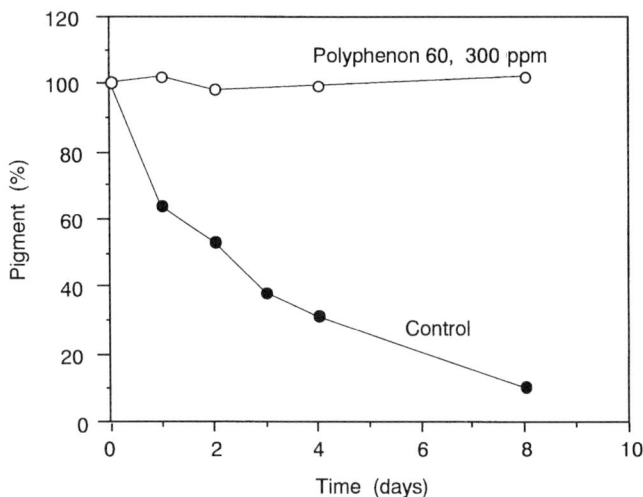

FIG. 9 Inhibition of deterioration of β-carotene by Polyphenon 60 (<60% green tea catechins).

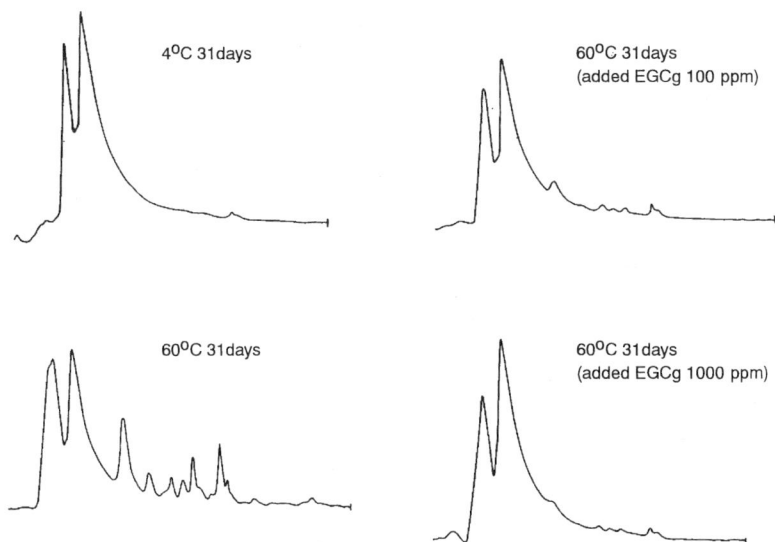

FIG. 10 Antioxidant effect of EGCg on D-limonene.

tion containing catechins (100 ppm) showed no change in color after five days while in the same time period the fish treated without catechins showed considerable discoloration.

C. Suppression of Oxidation of Natural Flavors

The effect of EGCg on limonene, the main component of lemon oil, was investigated (3). When D-limonene was kept for 31 days at 60°C, peaks of the oxidized products of limonene were observed. However, when EGCg in a concentration of 100 ppm was added, oxidation of limonene was almost completely suppressed (Fig. 10).

REFERENCES

1. T Matsuzaki, Y Hara. Antioxidative action of tea leaf catechins. Nippon Nogeikagaku Kaishi 59:129–134, 1985.
2. Y Hara. Prophylactic functions of tea polyphenols. In: CT Ho, T Osawa, MT Huang, R Rosen, ed. Food Phytochemicals for Can-

cer Prevention II, Teas Spices and Herbs. ACS Symposium Series 547:Am Chem Soc, 1994, pp 34–50.

3. Y Hara. Process for Production of Tea Catechins. U.S. Patent No.: 4,613,672, 1986.

4. F Nanjo, M Honda, K Okushio, N Matsumoto, F Ishigaki, T Ishigami, Y Hara. Effects of dietary catechins on α-tocopherol levels, lipid peroxidation, and erythrocyte deformability in rats fed on high palm oil and perilla oil diets. Biol Pharm Bull 16:1156–1159, 1993.

5. Y Hara. Process for the Production of a Natural Antioxidant Obtained from Tea Leaves. U.S. Patent No.: 4,673,530, 1987.

6

Radical Scavenging Action

I. INTRODUCTION

Free radicals are molecules that possess unpaired electrons. These molecules are in a constant state of instability for pairing with electrons and therefore are highly reactive with other molecules or compounds. Oxygen radicals such as super oxide anion radical ($O_2{}^\bullet-$), singlet oxygen ($^1O_2$), and hydroxyl radical ($^\bullet OH$) in particular, are inevitably generated in our body during the process of perspiration (metabolism) and are highly reactive with surrounding compounds. Not only do they react with lipids to produce degenerative lipid peroxides, but they also attack DNA or other organic constituents to induce various oxidative damage. These reactions inside the body are considered to be one of the irreversible causes of various diseases and aging. Radical oxygens and the resultant lipid peroxides in foods and in cosmetics are also detrimental to our health. The generation of radical oxygens and their actions, defense systems against them, the role of antioxidative flavonoids in relation to aging and diseases have been researched in great detail (1).

41

II. SCAVENGING EFFECTS OF CATECHINS ON DPPH RADICAL

We have determined the radical scavenging ability of tea catechins, their epimers and the derivatives with DPPH (1,1-diphenyl-2-picrylhydrazyl) radical, using electron spin resonance spectrometry (ESR) (2,3). Tea catechins and their epimers were shown to have 50% radical scavenging ability in the concentration range of 1 to 3 µM (Table 1). There were no significant differences observed between the scavenging activity of tea catechins and their epimers, and hence the scavenging effects of catechins are not dependent on their sterical structure. In order to identify the responsible groups in the catechins' structure, various acylated or glucosylated catechins underwent the same process as above.

TABLE 1 Scavenging Effects of Tea Catechins and Their Epimers on DPPH Radical

Galloyl group (G)

Catechins	Configuration	R1	R2	SC$_{50}$ (mM)
(+)-Epicatechin	2S, 3R	OH	H	2.9
(+)-Catechin	2R, 3S	OH	H	2.9
(−)-Epicatechin	2R, 3R	OH	H	3.0
(−)-Catechin	2S, 3R	OH	H	2.7
(−)-Epigallocatechin	2R, 3R	OH	OH	1.8
(−)-Gallocatechin	2S, 3R	OH	H	2.1
(−)-Epicatechin gallate	2R, 3R	G	H	1.2
(−)-Catechin gallate	2S, 3R	G	H	1.4
(−)-Epigallocatechin gallate	2R, 3R	G	OH	1.2
(−)-Gallocatechin gallate	2S, 3R	G	OH	1.1
α-Tocopherol (Vitamin E)				18
Ascorbic acid (Vitamin C)				13

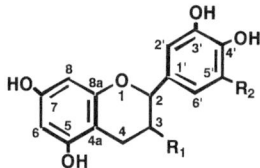

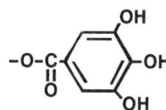

Table 2 shows the scavenging activity of acylated catechins. The scavenging effects of (+)-Catechin ((+)-C) were reduced drastically by the acetylation of hydroxyl groups in the B ring (3′, 4′-OH) whereas there was hardly any decrease in effectiveness with the modification of hydroxyl groups in the A ring (5, 7- or 3, 5, 7-OH). Specific acylation of the hydroxyl group of (+)-C or (−)-EGC at 3 position also caused no significant changes in activity. Thus, it is suggested that the A ring does not function as an advantageous structure to radical scavenging and that the presence of hydroxyl groups in the B ring is the important structural feature for radical scavenging ability.

TABLE 2   Scavenging Abilities of Partially Acylated Catechins on DPPH Radical

Compounds	SC_{50} (mM)
(+)-Catechin	2.4
(+)-Catechin 5,7-di-O-acetate (1)	1.3
(+)-Catechin 3,5,7-tri-O-acetate (2)	1.4
(+)-Catechin 3,3′,4′-tri-O-acetate (3)	>100
(+)-Catechin 5,7,3′,4′-tetra-O-acetate (4)	80
(−)-Catechin 3-O-acetate (5)	3.8
(−)-Catechin 3-O-propionate (6)	3.7
(−)-Epigallocatechin	1.8
(−)-Epigallocatechin 3-O-acetate (7)	2.1
(−)-Epigallocatechin 3-O-propionate (8)	2.0

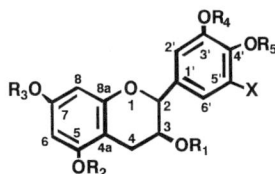

(1): R_1 = H, R_2 = R_3 = $COCH_3$, R_4 = R_5 = H, X = H
(2): R_1 = R_2 = R_3 = $COCH_3$, R_4 = R_5 = H, X = H
(3): R_1 = $COCH_3$, R_2 = R_3 = H, R_4 = R_5 = $COCH_3$, X = H
(4): R_1 = H, R_2 = R_3 = R_4 = R_5 = $COCH_3$, X = H
(5): R_1 = $COCH_3$, R_2 = R_3 = R_4 = R_5 = H, X = H
(6): R_1 = $COCH_2CH_3$, R_2 = R_3 = R_4 = R_5 = H, X = H
(7): R_1 = $COCH_3$, R_2 = R_3 = R_4 = R_5 = H, X = OH
(8): R_1 = $COCH_2CH_3$, R_2 = R_3 = R_4 = R_5 = H, X = OH

Table 3 shows the scavenging ability of some glucosylated catechins on the DPPH radical in comparison with that of the original catechins. Glucosylation at either 3′ or 4′ position (B ring) of (−)-EC, caused a marked decrease in scavenging ability. In the glycosides of (−)-EGC, with *ortho*-trihydroxyl group in its B ring, glucosylation at 4′ position markedly reduced

TABLE 3   Scavenging Abilities of Tea Catechin Glucosides on DPPH Radical

Compounds	SC_{50} (mM)
(−)-Epicatechin	2.4
(−)-Epicatechin 3′-Glc (9)	17
(−)-Epicatechin 4′-Glc (10)	21
(−)-Epigallocatechin	1.7
(−)-Epigallocatechin 3′-Glc (11)	3.1
(−)-Epigallocatechin 4′-Glc (12)	21
(−)-Epigallocatechin 3′,7-Glc (13)	4.7
(−)-Epicatechin gallate	1.1
(−)-Epicatechin gallate 3′-Glc (14)	1.0
(−)-Epigallocatechin gallate	1.2
(−)-Epigallocatechin gallate 3′-Glc (15)	1.0
(−)-Epigallocatechin gallate 4′-Glc (16)	1.8
(−)-Epigallocatechin gallate 7,3′-Glc (17)	1.2
(−)-Epigallocatechin gallate 4′,4″-Glc (18)	22

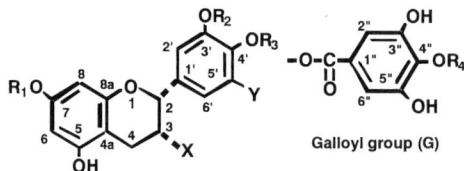

Galloyl group (G)

(9): X = OH, Y = H, R₁ = H, R₂ = Glc, R₃ = H
(10): X = OH, Y = H, R₁ = R₂ = H, R₃ = Glc
(11): X = OH, Y = OH, R₁ = H, R₂ = Glc, R₃ = H
(12): X = OH, Y = OH, R₁ = R₂ = H, R₃ = Glc
(13): X = OH, Y = OH, R₁ = R₂ = Glc, R₃ = H
(14): X = G, Y = H, R₁ = H, R₂ = Glc, R₃ = H, R₄ = H
(15): X = G, Y = OH, R₁ = H, R₂ = Glc, R₃ = H, R₄ = H
(16): X = G, Y = OH, R₁ = R₂ = H, R₃ = Glc, R₄ = H
(17): X = G, Y = OH, R₁ = R₂ = Glc, R₃ = H, R₄ = H
(18): X = G, Y = OH, R₁ = R₂ = H, R₃ = Glc, R₄ = Glc

scavenging ability, whereas that of 3' position reduced scavenging ability only slightly. Thus, it can be said that in free catechins, as well as in other flavonoids, the presence of an ortho-dihydroxyl group in the B ring is essential for realization of the scavenging ability and that ortho-trihydroxyls render scavenging ability even more effective. Scavenging ability seems to be further stabilized with galloyl moeties ((−)-ECg and (−)-EGCg). As shown in Table 3, even the glucosylation at 3' position for (−)-ECg or 4' position for (−)-EGCg will not reduce scavenging ability, while those for (−)-EC or (−)-EGC rendered them ineffective. These results show that the galloyl moiety at 3 position has a strong scavenging ability, equal or superior to the ortho-trihydroxyl group in the B ring. The glucosylation at 4' position (in the galloyl moiety) in addition to 4' position of EGCg caused significant loss in scavenging activity, indicating that meta-hydroxylation in the galloyl moiety, as well as in the B ring, has an unfavorable influence on the ability to scavenge the DPPH radical.

III. pH DEPENDENCY OF CATECHINS ON DPPH RADICAL

The effects of pH on the scavenging activity of tea catechins on the DPPH radical were examined. As shown in Table 4, the scavenging action of catechins was found to decline with decreasing pH value. Particularly, free catechins of ortho-dihydroxyls at B ring ((+)-C or (−)-EC) decreased in their scavenging ability markedly from pH 7 to 4. However, (−)-EGC with ortho-trihydroxyl structure were nearly ten times more potent than the dihydroxyls catechins at pH 4 and their effect was hardly affected by pH. The pH dependency of (−)-ECg and (−)-EGCg on scavenging ability was similar to that of (−)-EGC. These results suggest that the ortho-trihydroxyl group in the B ring and the galloyl moiety contribute to maintaining the DPPH radical scavenging ability more effectively at lower pH and that the scavenging efficiency of the ortho-dihydroxyl group in the B ring is limited in neutral and alka-

TABLE 4   Redox Potentials and DPPH Radical
Scavenging Abilities of (+)-Catechin and
(−)-Epigallocatechin at Different pH Values

	(+)-Catechin		(−)-Epigallocatechin	
	Ei (V)	SC$_{50}$ (nM)	Ei (V)	SC$_{50}$ (nM)
pH 4	0.74[b]	25	0.59[d]	3.3
pH 7	0.57[a]	2.4	0.42[c]	1.1
pH 10	0.47[b]	0.7	0.32[d]	0.9

[a] From Ref. 20.
[b] Calculated using the formula, $E_i = E_0 + 0.059 \log (Ka + 10^{-i})$,
from Ref. 40. pKa = 8.64 from Ref. 20.
[c] From Ref. 16.
[d] Calculated in the same manner as described in [b]. $E_7 = 0.42$ for
(−)-epigallocatechin. pKa = 8.71 for robinetinidol (7, 3′, 4′, 5′-
tetrahydroxyflavan-3-*ol*).

line conditions. Ariga et al. have reported that the antioxidant
activity of procyanidin B-3 ((+)-C dimer) is significantly
weaker in acidic conditions (pH 3–5) than at neutral or
slightly alkaline regions (pH 7–9) in linoleic acid–β-carotene–
water system (4). Their results are conceivable from our data
since procyanidins lack the *ortho*-trihydroxyl groups.

IV. COMPARISON OF RADICAL SCAVENGING POTENCY AND ANTIOXIDATIVITY OF POLYPHENON 60, PINE BARK OPC, AND GRAPE SEED OPC

Oligomeric proanthocyanidins (OPC) are catechin oligomers
found in a specific pine bark or in grape seed and are said
to have marked antioxidative potency as effected as radical
scavengers. The radical scavenging potency and antioxidativity of OPCs were compared with those of Polyphenon 60™,
a tea catechin mixture of more than 60% catechin content.

The results, as detailed in Chapter 19, showed by far
higher radical scavenging velocity and potency of Polyphenon
60 than pine bark OPC or grape seed OPC. In addition, Poly-

phenon 60 showed antioxidative effect in heated salad oil (120°C, 20 ml/min aeration), while there was no effect in the OPCs.

V. IN VIVO EXPERIMENT

Furukawa et al. irradiated x-rays to the larvae of *Drosophila melanogaster* in order to induce somatic cell mutations to be expressed as mutant spots on the wings of the hatched flies (5). The numbers of mutant spots of those flies, fed EGCg, EGC, or TF3 (theaflavin digallate) during the period of larvae, were significantly fewer as compared with those fed no tea polyphenols. In this experimental system, x-ray irradiation generated hydroxyl and other radicals that caused damage to the cellular DNA. Thus, tea polyphenols were confirmed by oral intake to suppress the chromosomal mutations caused by x-ray induced oxyradicals.

REFERENCES

1. CA Rice-Evans, L Packer, ed. Flavonoids in Health and Disease. New York: Marcel Dekker, 1998.
2. F Nanjo, K Goto, R Seto, M Suzuki, M Sakai, Y Hara. Scavenging effects of tea catechins and their derivatives on 1,1-diphenyl-2-picryhydrazyl radical. Free Radical Biol and Med 21:895–902, 1996.
3. F Nanjo, M Mori, K Goto, Y Hara. Radical scavenging activity of tea catechins and their related compounds. Biosci Biotechnol Biochem 63:1621–1623, 1999.
4. T Ariga, I Koshiyama, D Fukushima. Antioxidative properties of procyanidins B-1 and B-3 from azuki beans in aqueous system. Agric Biol Chem 52:2717–2722, 1988.
5. K Kawai, K Fujikawa, H Furukawa. Suppression of Genotoxicity or x-rays in somatic cells of *Drosophila melanogaster* by (−)-epigallocatechin gallate, (−)-epigallocatechin and theaflavin digallate. Envir Mut Res 21:103–107, 1999.

7

Antibacterial Action

I. INTRODUCTION

It seems that prescribing a cup of tea for an upset stomach can no longer be regarded as merely an old-fashioned remedy. Some people may remember being served up cups of tea to treat a bad cold or flu. Although it cannot be called a miracle cure, there is now some scientific data to support the idea that tea can have a calming effect when bacterial infections are present. People all over the world drink tea, and many cultures appear to have incorporated it into various customs. In Japan, green tea traditionally accompanies almost every meal, and particularly strong green tea is always drunk after eating sushi. Somehow, it seems that people have always known that tea can fight bacteria.

The antibacterial action of tea is attributed to the polyphenolic components it contains. It could potentially be exploited at all different levels: from protection of bacterial infection on an individual basis by consumption of polyphenols to the large-scale commercial use of polyphenols in order to prevent contamination of food products by pathogenic bacteria.

II. FOODBORNE PATHOGENIC BACTERIA

The polyphenolic components of tea have been found to be extremely effective against various strains of foodborne pathogenic bacteria that can be harmful and, in some incidences, even fatal (1). Food poisoning has claimed many lives in the past, and it is impossible to tell when or where it will crop up again, although it most certainly will. Tea polyphenols have shown an antibacterial effect against a number of such destructive bacteria, namely: *Clostridium perfringens, Vibrio parahaemolyticus, Vibrio fluvialis, Vibrio metchnikovii, Staphylococcus aureus, Bacillus cereus, Plesiomonas shigelloides,* and *Aeromonas sobria.* Such an immediate susceptibility was not seen with bacteria such as *Aeromonas hydrophila* subsp. *hydrophila, Salmonella enteritidis, Salmonella typhimurium,* enteropathogenic *Escherichia coli,* enteroinvasive *E. coli, Yersinia enterocolitica, Campylobacter jejuni,* and *Campylobacter coli,* although they were inhibited after a longer period of contact with tea polyphenols. The minimum inhibitory concentration was determined and is shown in Table 1.

III. THE FATE OF *Clostridium botulinum* SPORES IN CANNED TEA DRINKS

Heat tolerant bacteria, in particular *Clostridium botulinum,* which can be deadly, are a great concern in the canning industry. *C. botulinum* thrives in a low-acidic environment (pH 4.6 or above), which corresponds with the conditions of canned tea drinks. The spores of *C. botulinum* are, in effect, very heat tolerant. When the spores germinate to grow to vegetative bacteria, they produce toxins. The botulinum toxin is deadly and kills half of 1 billion mice at a concentration of 1 mg of nitrogen in the toxin (10^9ip LD_{50} mice/1mg-N, S toxin). Lethal dose for a human is considered to be a few µg. Therefore, it is the responsibility of the food canning industry to kill the spores of

TABLE 1 Minimum Inhibitory Concentrations of Catechins and Theaflavins Against Foodborne Pathogenic Bacteria

Bacteria	MIC (ppm)									
	GTC	EC	ECg	EGC	EGCg	CTFs	TF1	TF2A	TF2B	TF3
Staphylococcus aureus IAM 1011	450	>800	800	150	250	500	500	400	150	200
Vibrio fluvialis JCM 3752	200	800	300	300	200	400	500	500	400	500
V. parahaemolyticus IFO 12711	200	800	500	300	200	300	300	500	400	500
V. metschnikovii IAM 1039	500	>1000	>1000	500	1000	300	600	800	700	800
Clostridium perfringens JCM 3816	400	>1000	400	1000	300	200	500	600	500	400
Bacillus cereus JCM 2152	600	>1000	600	>1000	600	500	600	1000	1000	800
Plesiomonas shigelloides IID No. 3	100	700	100	200	100	100	200	200	200	100
Aeromonas sobria JCM 2139	400	>1000	700	400	300	300	600	600	400	500

GTC, green tea catechins
CTFs, crude theaflavins

this bacteria. Billions of spores/ml are confirmed to be killed by heating at 121°C for 4 min. Over the last 10 years or so canned tea has been a growing market in Japan, with this popularity recently starting to spread to the United States and other countries. Present health regulations dictate strict rules for sterilization under which the spores of *C. botulinum* are without doubt eliminated. The product must, theoretically, be heated at 121°C for at least 4 min. However, this severe heating process has a detrimental effect on the quality of the product, resulting in a poorer taste and aroma of the tea. A practical alternative is to heat the canned product at 130°C or over for at least a few seconds, which is more than the equivalent energy expended in the case of treatment at 121°C for 4 min. Either way, the flavor of canned tea is inferior to a product that undergoes a more mild heat treatment.

Thus, if *C. botilinum* spores could be eliminated without employing such drastic heating for sterilization, it would be of great advantage to the industry. Accordingly, in view of tea's antibacterial actions, some investigations were carried out into the fate of *C. botulinum* in canned tea beverages (2). Green tea, oolong tea, and two kinds of black teas—sweetened (8% sugar) and lightly sweetened (5% sugar)—were inoculated with *C. botulinum* spores (type A and type B, composed of a mixture of 5 strains each) to the concentration of about 500 spores/ml and incubated for 30 days at 30°C , without any heat treatment after inoculation. The viable countings were calculated by most probable number (MPN) method and pouch method. (MPN is a method for counting the number of spores in the solution by diluting the test solution decimally until a certain dilution does not kill the mice by intraperitoneal [ip] injection. From the number of this dilution the number of spores in the initial solution is determined. With the pouch method, the test solution is inoculated into the medium, the spores grow anaerobically, and the number of colonies are counted in the flat pouch.) In all of the tea drinks except green tea, there was a marked decrease in the viable cell count (Fig. 1). In the case of green tea, subsequent heating of the inocu-

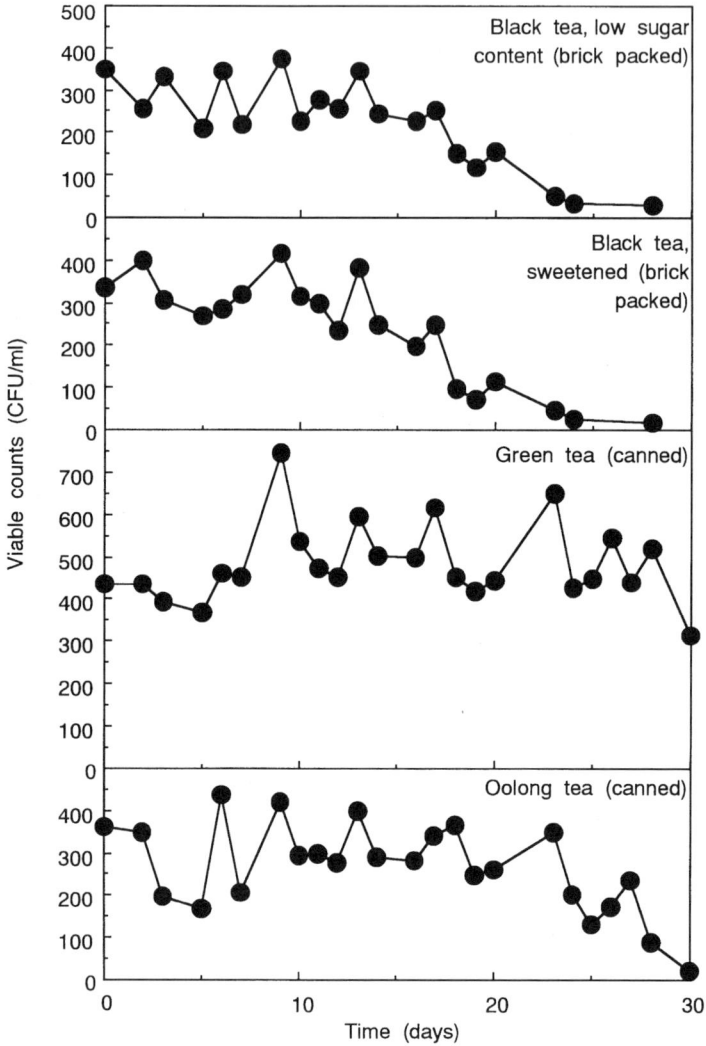

FIG. 1 Changes in *C. botulinum* spore numbers after inoculation into various kinds of tea drinks without heat treatment.

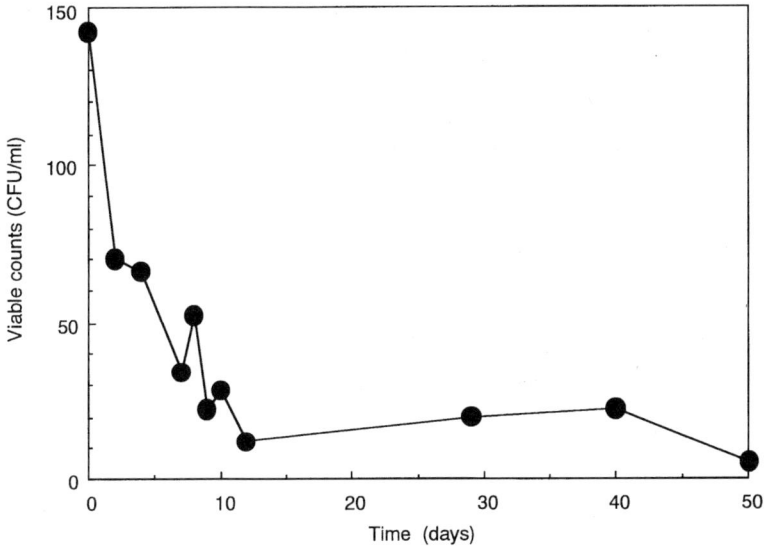

FIG. 2 Changes in *C. botulinum* spore numbers after inoculation into canned green tea with treatment for 30 min at 85°C.

lated liquid for 30 minutes at 85°C decreased the viable spores (Fig. 2). In order to determine what components of the tea were responsible for the inhibition of spore proliferation, the polyphenolic and nonpolyphenolic fractions were isolated and each was incubated respectively with *C. botulinum*. The polyphenolic fraction was confirmed to be effective as indicated by a decrease in the viable spore count, while the non-polyphenolic fraction had no inhibitory influence on the spore count (Fig. 3).

IV. ANTIBACTERIAL ACTIVITY OF TEA POLYPHENOLS AGAINST *C. botulinum* AND OTHER HEAT TOLERANT BACTERIA

In the previous experiment, the fate of *C. botulinum* spores inoculated into tea drinks was examined. It was confirmed that the polyphenolic component of tea drinks killed the spores as well as the vegetative cells of *C. botulinum*. Pursu-

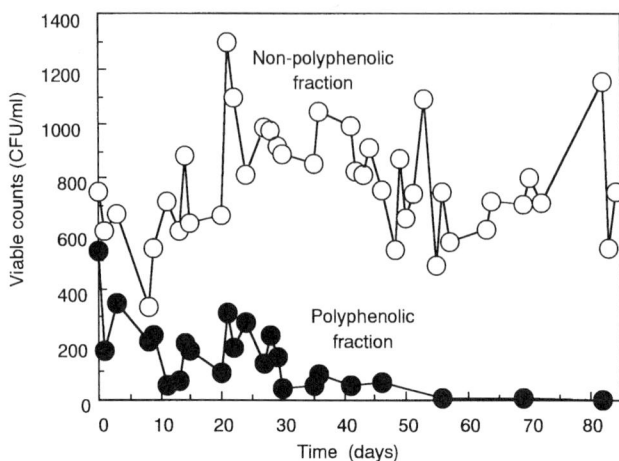

FIG. 3 Changes in *C. botulinum* spore numbers after inoculation into the polyphenolic fractions from black tea.

ant to the above, minimum inhibitory concentration (MIC) of each tea polyphenolic component against spores of *C. botulinum* was determined (3). The constituents of the polyphenolic fraction of green tea (GTC) and black tea (crude theaflavins) are described in Chapter 4. The MIC of these fractions

TABLE 2 MIC of Tea Polyphenols Against *C. botulinum* (ppm)

	Spores	Vegetative cells
GTC	300	<100
EGC	>1000	300
EC	>1000	>1000
EGCg	200	<100
ECg	200	200
Crude theaflavins	200	200
TF1	250	150
TF2 (A&B)	150	250
TF2A	150	250
TF2B	150	150
TF3	100	200

TABLE 3 MIC of Tea Polyphenols Against *B. subtilis*, *B. stearothermophilus*, and *D. nigrificans* (ppm)

	B. subtilis		*B. stearothermophilus*		*D. nigrificans*	
	Spores	Vegetative cells	Spores	Vegetative cells	Spores	Vegetative cells
GTC	>1000	>800	300	200	<100	>1000
EGC	>1000	>800	1000	300	500	>1000
EC	>1000	>800	>1000	800	500	>1000
EGCg	1000	>800	200	200	200	>1000
ECg	900	>800	300	<100	<100	>1000
Crude theaflavins	600	700	300	200	<100	>1000
TF1	>500	>1000	250	200	200	>1000
TF2 (A&B)	—	—	200	—	100	—
TF2A	>500	500	—	300	—	>1000
TF2B	500	450	—	300	—	>1000
TF3	400	400	150	200	100	>1000

and their individual components against the spores and the vegetative cells of *C. botulinum* is shown in Table 2. Even the resistant spores were killed at concentrations of 200–300 ppm. These data support the antibotulinum potency of canned teas; in ordinary tea drinks, polyphenolic components are contained somewhere from 500–1,000 ppm. Furthermore, the MIC of these tea polyphenols was examined against such heat resistant bacteria as *Bacillus subtilis*, *B. stearothermophilus*, and *Desulfotomaculum nigrificans* as shown in Table 3. These data indicate that (a) tea polyphenols show almost the same antibacterial potency against the most representative "flat sour" bacteria *B. stearothermophilus* as against *C. botulinum*, (b) tea polyphenols did not work against *B. subtilis* as effectively as against *B. stearothermophilus*, and (c) tea polyphenols were effective against the spores but not against the vegetative cells of *D. nigrificans*, a common putrefactive bacteria in fish cans. These results revealed that the antibacterial spectrum of tea polyphenols is random and unpredictable.

REFERENCES

1. Y Hara, T Ishigami. Antibacterial activities of tea polyphenols against foodborne pathogenic bacteria (studies on antibacterial effects of tea polyphenols part III) [in Japanese]. Nippon Shokuhin Kogyo Gakkaishi 36:996–999, 1989.
2. Y Hara, M Watanabe. The fate of *Clostridium botulinum* spores inoculated into tea drinks (studies on antibacterial effects of tea polyphenols part I) [in Japanese]. Nippon Shokuhin Kogyo Gakkaishi 36:375–379, 1989.
3. Y Hara, M Watanabe. Antibacterial activity of tea polyphenols against *Clostridium botulinum* (studies on antibacterial effects of tea polyphenols part II) [in Japanese]. Nippon Shokuhin Kogyo Gakkaishi 36:951–955, 1989.

8

Methicillin-Resistant
Staphylococcus aureus

I. INTRODUCTION

Methicillin-resistant *Staphylococcus aureus* (MRSA) is currently a serious problem in hospitals, where patients with lowered resistance are at considerable risk. *S. aureus* is a very common bacterium that causes bacterium-infectious diseases. It is normally present in the environment and resides in the affected purulent area of inflammation, the skin, nose, and pharynx. Since this bacterium produces exotoxins and exoenzymes, the bacterium has highly pathogenic properties and is the cause of various diseases, such as infectious diseases of the skin and flesh, infectious diseases of the intestinal tracts (food poisoning), septicemia, endocarditis, cerebromeningitis, infectious diseases of the respiratory organs, and infectious diseases of the urinary passages. As long as the host is resistant enough, there will not be any proliferation of the bacteria nor any occurrence of infectious diseases. When there is an outbreak of infection, it has been routine practice to administer antibiotics in order to eliminate the bacteria and remedy the disease. However, the presence of a so-called antibiotic-resistant $S. aureus$ that is unaffected by administration of antibiotics is now known, and today it is prevalent particularly in clinical institutions where antibiotics are used profusely.

II. ANTI-MRSA ACTIVITY OF TEA POLYPHENOLS

Previously, we confirmed that tea polyphenols have an antibacterial action on SA ($S. aureus$) (1). Pursuant to this, we collaborated with Shimamura (2) and Kono (3) in investigating the antibacterial effect of (−)-epigallocatechin gallate (EGCg) or theaflavin digallate (TF3) on MRSA of clinical isolates. Results show very low minimum inhibitory concentrations for EGCg (32–64 μg/ml) or TF3 (125 μg/ml). Further, the bactericidal effect of EGCg when mixing it with a bacterial solution (10^4/ml) was confirmed by Shimamura et al. As shown in Fig. 1, at 250 μg(EGCg)/ml, no decline of survival counts was observed in the first three hours. After 24 hours, there was an apparent decrease in the count. At a concentration of 500 μg(EGCg)/ml, no bacterium survived after 24 hours of contact. Catechin concentration in a cup of green tea is about 500–1,000 μg/ml and more than half of it is composed of EGCg. These facts suggest that MRSA is susceptible to tea at a strength normally consumed.

Clinical trials with inpatients have been undertaken at the hospital at Fukuoka University, Medical School, Japan (unpublished data). MRSA, present in the nasal cavity and trachea of carriers who showed no apparent symptoms of infection, was identified on examination of their sputum. Most of the 23 patients were over 70 years old and had been admitted to hospital for treatment of various ailments. They were given an inhalation containing tea catechins (Polyphenon 100, catechins >90%). Catechins were dissolved in 10 ml of saline or bromohexine and administered with a nebulizer 2–3 times a day.

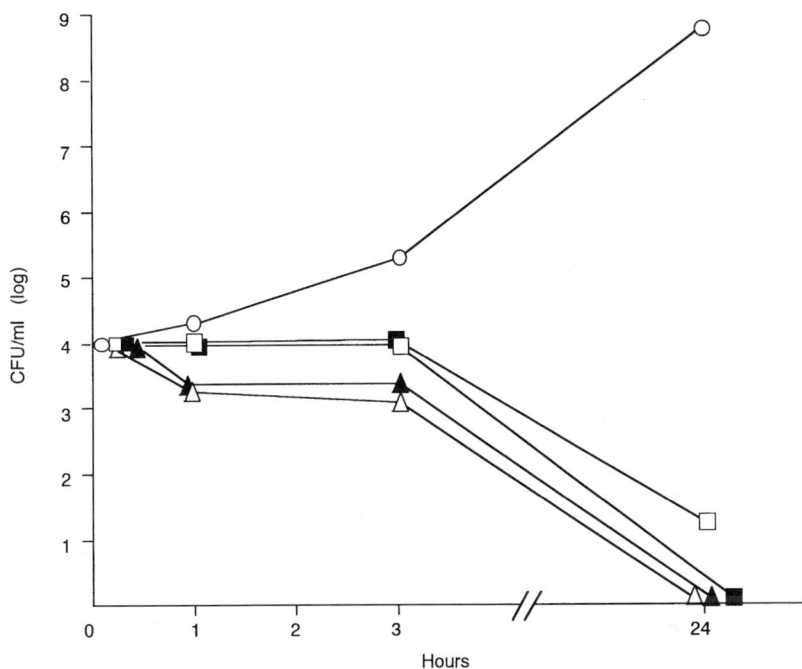

FIG. 1 Bactericidal activity of tea extract and EGCg against MRSA (H5). (O) control; (△) 2.5% black tea; (▲) 5% black tea; (□) 250 µg/ml EGCg; (■) 500 µg/ml EGCg.

Inhalation of 20–40 mg catechins per day appeared to eliminate MRSA but there was a recurrence. A dose of 80 mg/day was effective without any incidence of reoccurrence. It took an average of six days to eliminate the bacteria and a 10 day follow-up confirmed the elimination of MRSA.

III. REVITALIZATION OF ANTIBIOTICS WITH TEA POLYPHENOLS

Antibiotics that show no antibacterial potency due to the resistance of the bacteria were found in in vitro tests to be revitalized with the addition of tea catechins (4). Shimamura et al. investigated the antibacterial potency of antibiotics, such as oxacillin (MPIPC), against MRSA in the presence of a concentration of tea catechins below minimum inhibitory concentration (MIC).

Green tea catechin (GTC, Polyphenon 100) at concentrations less than the MIC (which ranges 125–250 µg/ml against clinical MRSA strains) was dissolved in sterilized water and added in final concentrations of 25, 50, and 100 µg/ml to a melting Meuller-Hinton agar by keeping it at a temperature of 60°C. To 98 ml of this agar, 2 ml of Meuller-Hinton broth in which test bacteria had been cultivated for 18 hours was added and mixed well. Immediately thereafter, 10 ml each of the above was poured into the petri dish. After cooling, a stainless cup (φ 8 mm) was put on the agar plate in the dish and into the cup was poured 0.1 ml of each of the various dilutions of antibiotics. After refrigerating for an hour, they were cultured overnight in a 36°C incubator. The following day the size of the growth inhibition zone around the cup was measured by slide calipers. Results are shown in Figs. 2–10. The antibiotics used were oxacillin (Fig. 2), methicillin (Fig. 3), aminobenzyl penicillin (Fig. 4), cephalexin (Fig. 5), penicillin G (Fig. 6), amikacin (Fig. 7), tetracycline (Fig. 8), chloramphenicol (Fig. 9), and gentamicin (Fig. 10). In the figures, ○ indicates GTC at a concentration of 100 µg/ml, ● indicates GTC at a concentration of 50 µg/ml, □ indicates GTC at a concentration of 25 µg/ml, and ■ indicates the control containing no GTC. As is evident from these figures, under the cup method the clinical MRSA of this test strain showed resistance with up to 2000 µg/ml oxacillin, but when 25 µg/ml of GTC was added to the culture, oxacillin regained an antibacterial action at 10 µg/ml, and the size of the inhibition zone grew larger as the concentration of the antibiotic increased. This synergistic effect was more pronounced as the concentration of catechins increased from 25 to 100 µg/ml. In the same way, the synergistic effect of methicillin, aminobenzyl penicillin, cephalexin, penicillin G, i.e., β-lactams, was confirmed. Amikacin, tetracycline, and chloramphenicol also showed a synergistic effect, but that of gentamicin was low. We have confirmed that the principal

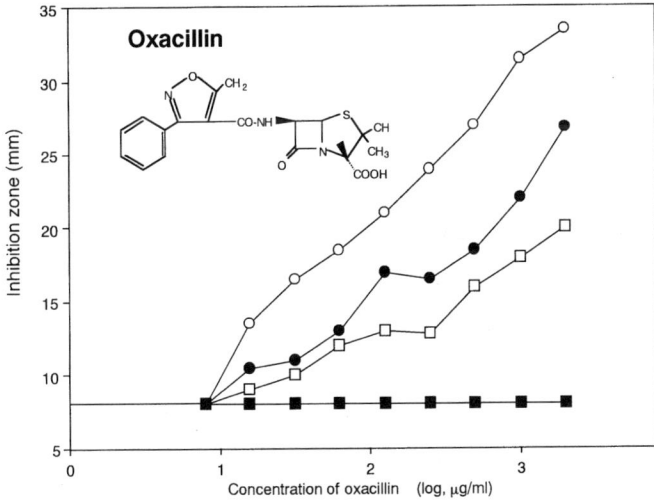

FIG. 2 Synergistic inhibitory effects of GTC and oxacillin on growth of MRSA. ─■─ GTC 0 µg/ml; ─□─ GTC 25 µg/ml; ─●─ GTC 50 µg/ml; ─○─ GTC 100 µg/ml.

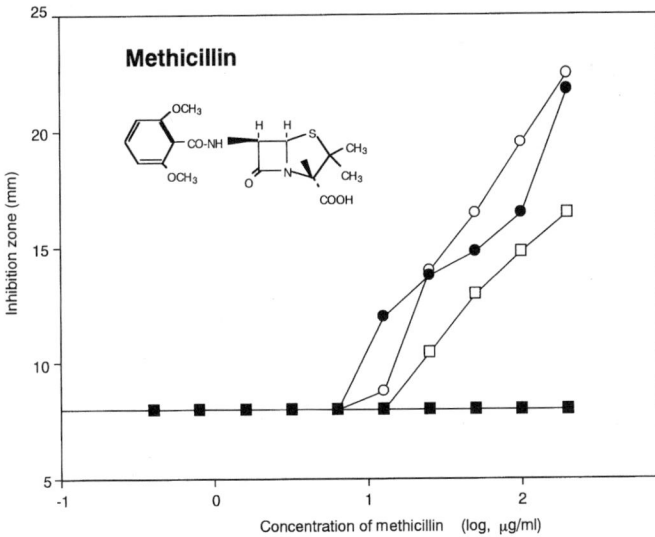

FIG. 3 Synergistic inhibitory effects of GTC and methicillin on growth of MRSA. ─■─ GTC 0 µg/ml; ─□─ GTC 25 µg/ml; ─●─ GTC 50 µg/ml; ─○─ GTC 100 µg/ml.

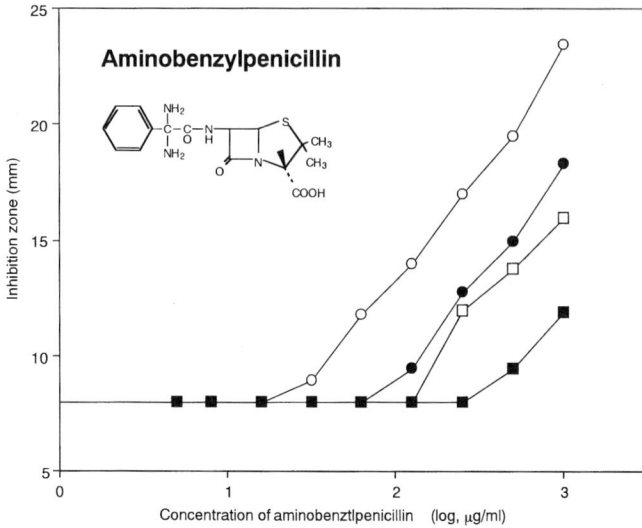

FIG. 4 Synergistic inhibitory effects of GTC and aminobenzylpenicillin on growth of MRSA. ─■─ GTC 0 μg/ml; ─□─ GTC 25 μg/ml; ─●─ GTC 50 μg/ml; ─○─ GTC 100 μg/ml.

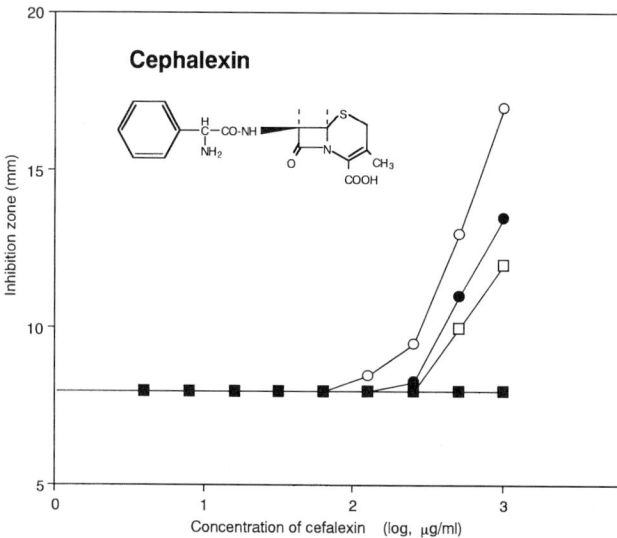

FIG. 5 Synergistic inhibitory effects of GTC and cephalexin on growth of MRSA. ─■─ GTC 0 μg/ml; ─□─ GTC 25 μg/ml; ─●─ GTC 50 μg/ml; ─○─ GTC 100 μg/ml.

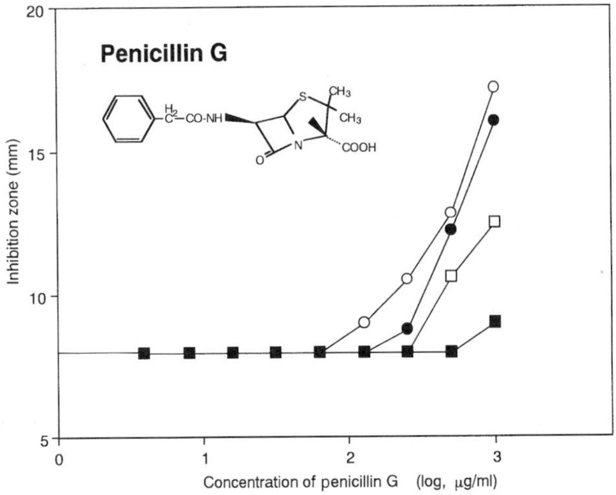

FIG. 6 Synergistic inhibitory effects of GTC and penicillin on growth of MRSA. ■— GTC 0 µg/ml; □— GTC 25 µg/ml; ●— GTC 50 µg/ml; ○— GTC 100 µg/ml.

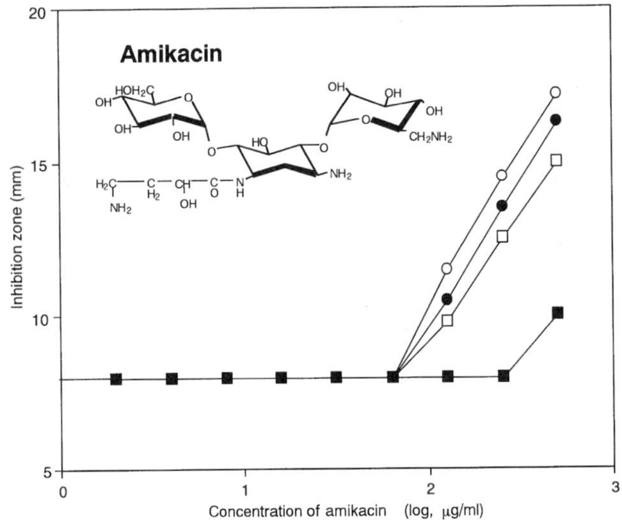

FIG. 7 Synergistic inhibitory effects of GTC and amikacin on growth of MRSA. ■— GTC 0 µg/ml; □— GTC 25 µg/ml; ●— GTC 50 µg/ml; ○— GTC 100 µg/ml.

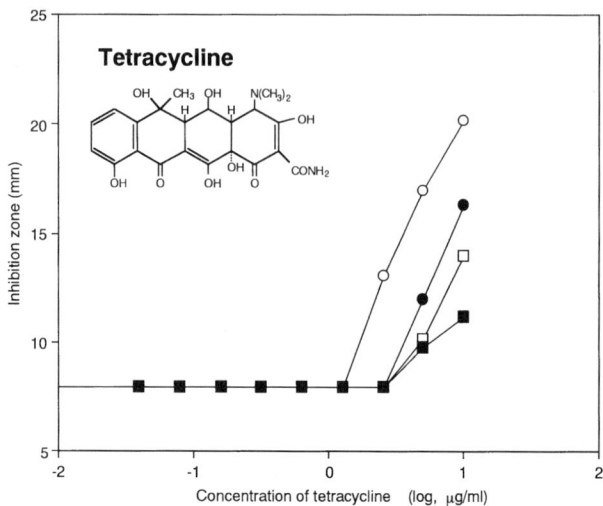

FIG. 8 Synergistic inhibitory effects of GTC and tetracycline on growth of MRSA. ■ GTC 0 μg/ml; □ GTC 25 μg/ml; ● GTC 50 μg/ml; ○ GTC 100 μg/ml.

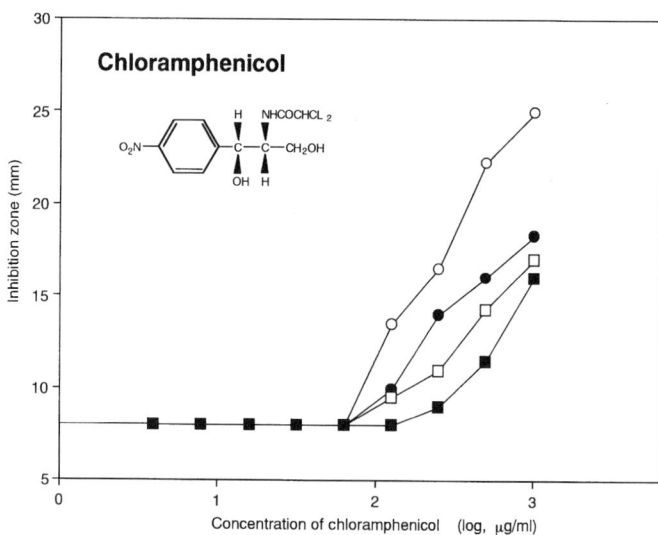

FIG. 9 Synergistic inhibitory effects of GTC and chloramphenicol on growth of MRSA. ■ GTC 0 μg/ml; □ GTC 25 μg/ml; ● GTC 50 μg/ml; ○ GTC 100 μg/ml.

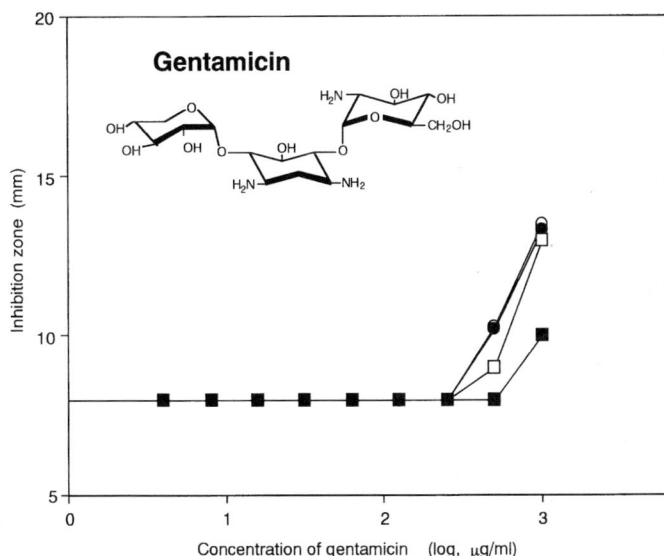

FIG. 10 Synergistic inhibitory effects of GTC and gentamicin on growth of MRSA. ─■─ GTC 0 µg/ml; ─□─ GTC 25 µg/ml; ─●─ GTC 50 µg/ml; ─○─ GTC 100 µg/ml.

components of these actions in GTC are such galloyl catechins as EGCg or ECg and not free catechins.

Curiously and notably, certain antibiotics show no antibacterial potency nor synergism with catechins against MRSA. Fig. 11 shows that kanamycin has no bactericidal effect against MRSA nor has any synergism with tea catechins. The same was confirmed with erythromycin, clindamycin, and colistin.

These facts have been noted by other researchers (5,6) and the underlying mechanisms were investigated. It seems that certain enzymes of MRSA are involved in the resistance formation and that the enzyme inhibitory property of tea polyphenols works specifically against them (7).

The emergence of antibiotic-resistant bacteria is a very grave threat to human and animal health care. When bacteria acquire resistance against certain antibiotics, and we are un-

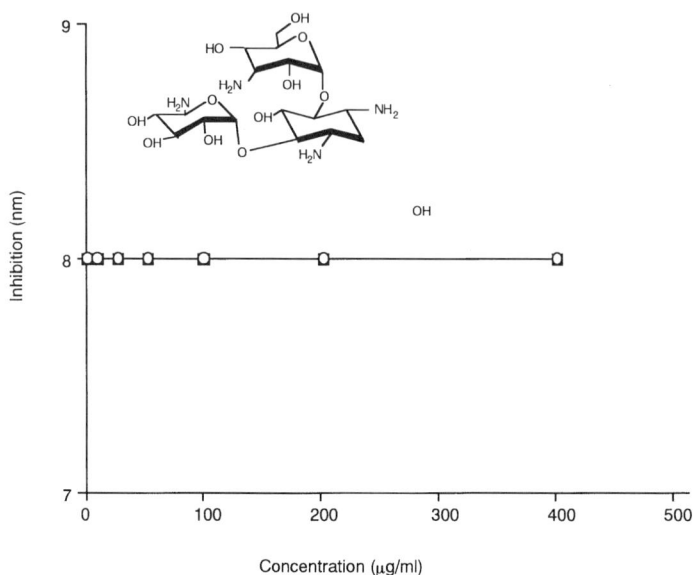

FIG. 11 Synergistic inhibitory effects of GTC and kanamycin on growth of MRSA. ■ GTC 0 µg/ml; □ GTC 25 µg/ml; ● GTC 50 µg/ml; ○ GTC 100 µg/ml.

able to find new effective ways to combat them, they will prevail and cause the emergence of various pathogenic and infectious diseases. The fact that tea catechins have the ability to revitalize the antibiotics that have lost potency against resistant bacteria has tremendous importance for the years to come, since so many antibiotics have been overused and are prone to bacterial resistance. Detailed studies on catechin–antibiotic synergism and their practical applications are underway.

REFERENCES

1. Y Hara, T Ishigami. Antibacterial activities of tea polyphenols against foodborne bacteria (studies on antibacterial effects of tea polyphenols part III) [in Japanese]. Nippon Shokuhin Kogyo Gakkaishi 36:996–999, 1989.

2. M Toda, S Okubo, Y Hara, T Shimamura. Antibacterial and bacterial activities of tea extracts and catechins against methicillin resistant *Staphylococcus aureus* [in Japanese]. Nihon Saikingaku Zasshi 46:839–845, 1991.
3. K Kono, I Tatara, S Takeda, K Arakawa, Y Hara. Antibacterial activity of epigallocatechin gallate against mechicillin-resistant *Staphylococcus aureus*. Kansenshougaku Zasshi 68:1518–1522, 1994.
4. O Takahashi, Z Cai, M Toda, Y Hara, T Shimamura. Appearance of antibacterial activity of oxacillin against methicillin resistant *Staphylococcus aureus* (MRSA) in the presence of catechin [in Japanese]. Kansenshougaku Zasshi 69:1126–1134, 1995.
5. Kureha Kagaku Kogyou Co., Ltd.: Japanese Patent Kokai No. 8-26991, 1996.
6. JMT Hamilton-Miller. U.S. Patent No. 5,879,683, 1999.12.20.
7. TS Yam, JMT Hamilton-Miller, S Shah. The effect of a component of tea (*Camellia sinensis*) on methicillin resistance, PBP2′ synthesis, and β-lactamase production in *Staphylococcus aureus*. J Antimicro Chemo 42:211–216, 1998.

9

Anticariogenic Action

I. INTRODUCTION

Dental caries are caused primarily by the bacterium *Strepto-coccus mutans,* which resides in the mouth and produces water-soluble and water-insoluble glucans from sucrose by cell-bound or extracellular glucosyltransferase. The insoluble glucan sticks to the surface of the tooth, and this is the beginning of plaque formation. Under the sticky glucan on the dental surface, *S. mutans* proliferates and, with a supply of sucrose, produces more glucans on the teeth. During the process of proliferation, *S. mutans* also produces lactic acid from sucrose, melting the enamel. This is the process of dental decay. Therefore, prevention of dental caries could be achieved by (a) suppressing the growth of *S. mutans*, (b) suppressing or destroying the formation of glucan (dental plaque), or (c) eating no sugar or food containing sugar. Tooth brushing is an effective method of removing dental plaque, which is the product and abode of *S. mutans*.

Tea polyphenols are anticarious in three ways: (a) They inhibit the plaque forming enzyme, (b) they suppress the growth of *S. mutans,* and (c) they solidify the enamel. These facts have come to light only recently. A relationship between tea and the prevention of dental caries has been previously considered since tea contains more fluoride than other plants and vegetables.

Separate research by Kashket in 1985 reported inhibition of glucosyltransferase by polyphenolic compounds in soft drinks (1). The suppression of the growth of *S. mutans* was also reported by S. Sakanaka et al. in 1989 (2).

II. EPIDEMIOLOGICAL STUDIES

Several epidemiological studies have investigated the benefits of tea drinking for the prevention of tooth decay. Onishi et al. were some of the first to conduct large-scale studies around 1972–1985 (3). They looked at the incidences of dental cavities among children in a tea-drinking program in two Japanese villages over a period of five years. The program consisted of the children drinking a cup of tea with their school lunch every day. About 100 ml of tea, which contained a relatively high amount of fluorine, was consumed. A reduction in the rate of carious lesions was noted. While this anticarious effect was attributed mainly to the fluorine content, it was recognized that other nonfluorine compounds contained in tea leaves are also effective.

Another study looked at the incidence of caries in primary and junior high school students of a tea-producing area in China (4). The mean caries incidence was discovered to be much lower than that of other areas in China, and the study concluded this was due to the well-established tea-drinking habit in that area. This study also investigated the benefits of fluoride, while additionally considering the role of tea catechins in preventing development of tooth caries by inhibition of the cariogenic bacteria *Streptococcus deformans,* and inhibition of the plaque forming process. The tea with the highest catechin content was found to be by far the most effective in inhibiting the growth, acidogenesis, and adhesion of *S. deformans*. This inhibiting effect increased in proportion to an increase in tea concentration.

III. INHIBITION OF PLAQUE FORMATION

The inhibition of the plaque-forming enzyme glucosyltransferase (GTF) by tea polyphenols was investigated in vitro (5). The enzyme GTF, sucrose, and tea polyphenols were mixed and incubated at 37°C for an hour. The sucrose carbon was labeled so that the fate of sucrose could be traced. Without tea poly-

TABLE 1 Effect of Tea Polyphenols on Insoluble-Glucan Formations Catalyzed by GTF (glucosyltransferase)

Sample	Concentration (mM)	% incorporation of (^{14}C) glucose[a] insoluble glucan
(−)-Catechin	1.0	77.7 ± 5.9[b]
	10.0	38.3 ± 3.0
(−)-Epicatechin	1.0	94.5 ± 3.5
	10.0	57.7 ± 5.0
(−)-Epicatechin gallate	1.0	64.5 ± 6.2
	10.0	17.0 ± 3.2
(−)-Gallocatechin gallate	1.0	52.8 ± 2.6
	10.0	4.6 ± 0.1
(−)-Epigallocatechin gallate	1.0	58.4 ± 3.3
	10.0	25.0 ± 1.9
(−)-Free theaflavin	1.0	43.2 ± 1.4
	10.0	1.7 ± 0.2
Theaflavin monogallate A	1.0	35.5 ± 1.6
	10.0	2.7 ± 0.6
Theaflavin monogallate B	1.0	52.9 ± 7.1
	10.0	2.2 ± 0.4
Theaflavin digallate	1.0	44.1 ± 2.6
	10.0	1.8 ± 0.3

[a] Incorporation ratios into insoluble-glucans relative to the respective control are expressed as follows: % incorporation = test (^{14}C-incorporation)/control (^{14}C-incorporation) ×100.
[b] Mean ± S.E. ($n = 4$).

phenols, the enzyme catalyzes the formation of insoluble glucan, i.e., plaque. In the solutions containing tea polyphenols
a dose-dependent inhibition of insoluble glucan formation was
noticeable. EGCg (and its isomer, GCg) and all theaflavins inhibited the glucan formation almost completely at the concentration of 10 mM. At 1 mM, about the drinking concentration
of tea polyphenols, more than 50% inhibition was observed
(Table 1).

Pursuant to the above, we have observed the influence of
tea beverages on the formation of plaque by *S. mutans*. The
method is described in Fig. 1. Tea leaves were drawn to make
a tea extract of normal concentration (2 g/200 ml hot water)
containing about 1,000 ppm of polyphenol concentration and

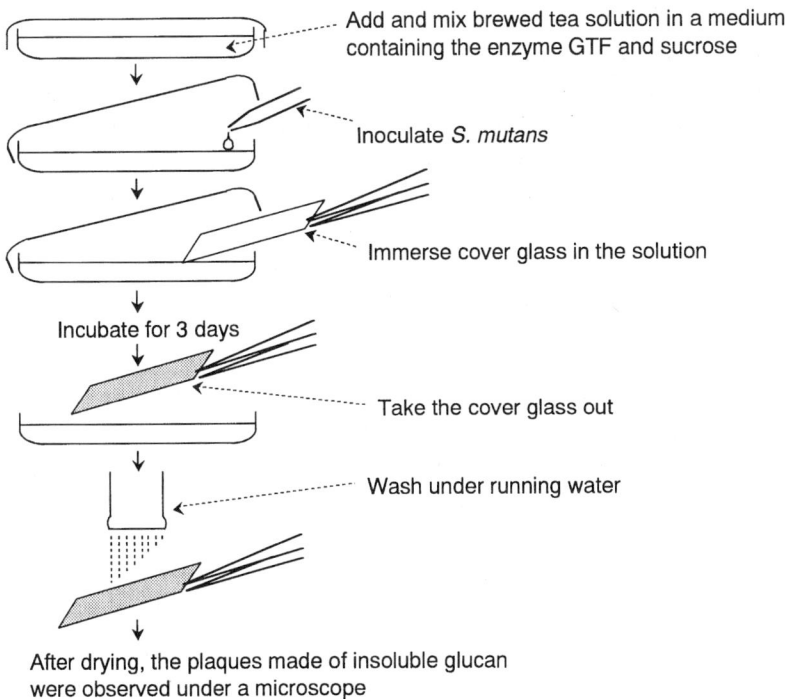

Add and mix brewed tea solution in a medium
containing the enzyme GTF and sucrose

Inoculate *S. mutans*

Immerse cover glass in the solution

Incubate for 3 days

Take the cover glass out

Wash under running water

After drying, the plaques made of insoluble glucan
were observed under a microscope

FIG. 1 Method for microscopic observation of dental plaques (insoluble glucan). GTF, glucosyltransferase.

thereafter diluted. Sucrose at 1% concentration was dissolved in the normal and the diluted brews. After adding drops of bacterial solution to the test beverage, a cover glass was immersed in the solution and incubated at 37°C for 3 days. The bacterial plaque formed on the surface of the cover glass was observed. All tea beverages (black tea, oolong tea, green tea, and puer tea) at normal concentrations and up to 4 times dilution were found to inhibit plaque formation (Fig. 2).

IV. INHIBITION OF THE PROLIFERATION OF
   S. mutans

We also confirmed the inhibitory potency of various tea beverages extracted at normal drinking concentrations on the growth of S. mutans. The results in Fig. 3 show that green tea is most effective in suppressing the growth of the bacteria. The separation of black tea infusion into polyphenolic and nonpolyphenolic fractions, which were adjusted to normal drinking concentration, acted on the bacteria as shown in Fig. 4. Polyphenolic fraction suppressed the growth of S. mutans, while the nonpolyphenolic fraction had no effect.

V. STRENGTHENING ACID RESISTANCY OF
   TEETH

It is known that tea contains 300–2000 ppm fluoride of which more than 50% is extracted into the tea infusion. Fluoride exists as fluoroapatite in the enamel of teeth, and it is well known that it strengthens the acid resistancy of the enamel. As a model for tooth decay, hydroxy apatite (HA), which has the same composition, as enamel, $Ca_5(OH)(PO_4)_3$, was used; and the acidic environment which is produced by lactic acid in the mouth was replaced by acetate buffer (pH 4) in this model.

Using the above model, Hayakawa et al. investigated acid resistance of HA with various components (6). First, the uptake of fluoride was measured by shaking 100 mg of HA with

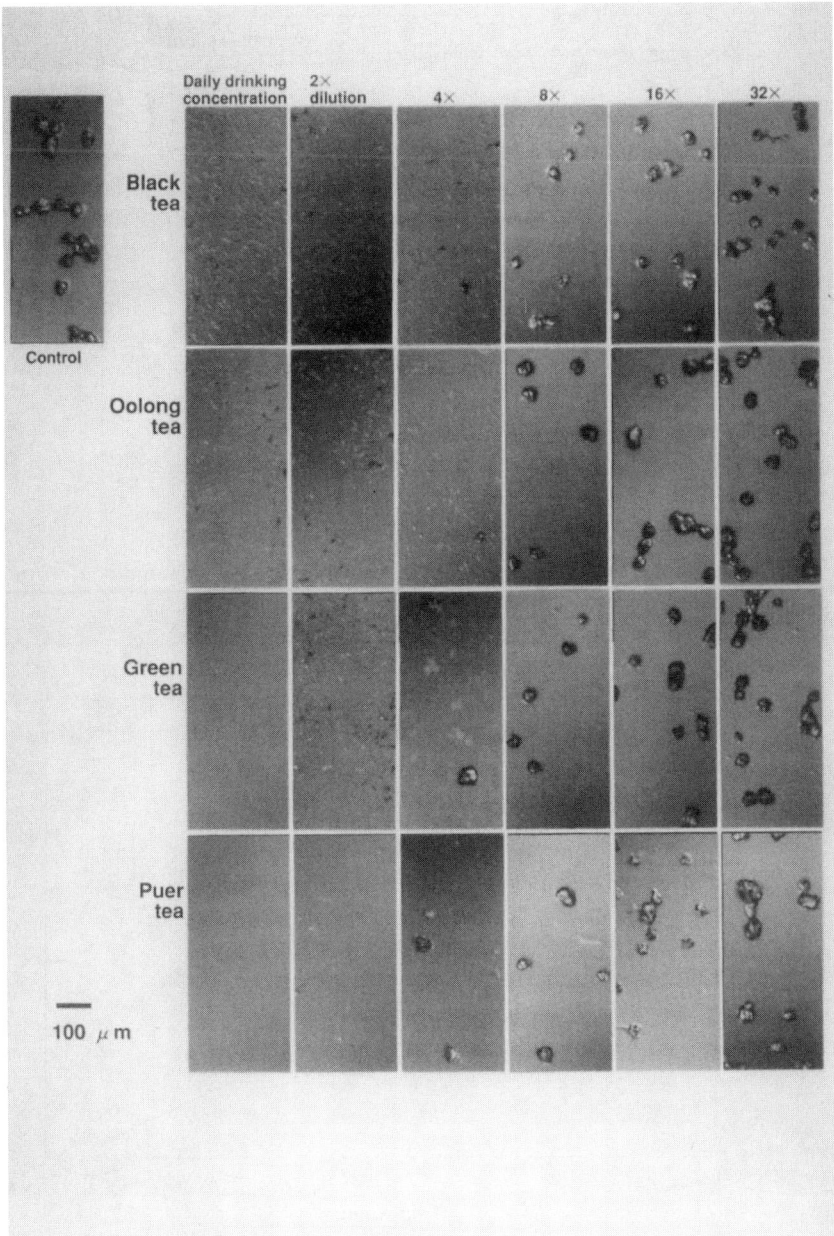

FIG. 2   Anti-dental plaque effect of tea beverages.

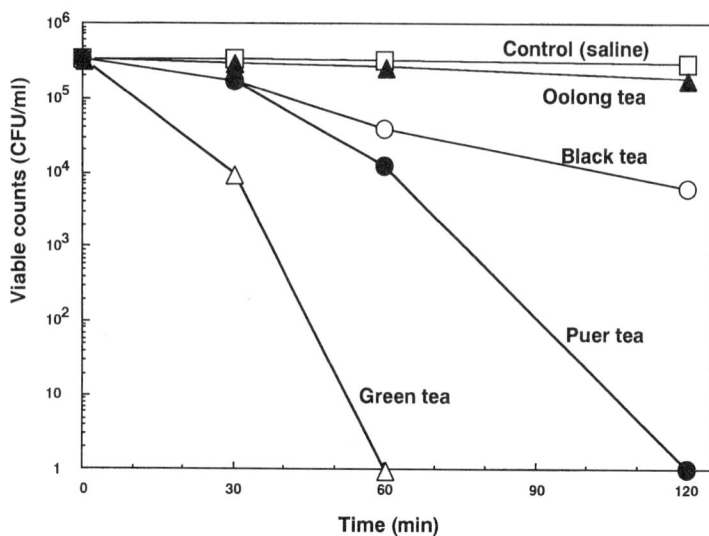

FIG. 3 Antibacterial effect of tea beverages against cariogenic bacterium *S. mutans.*

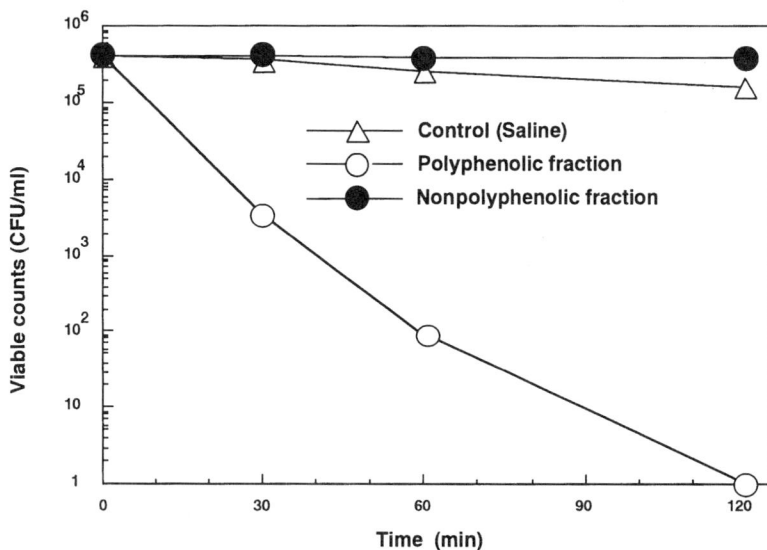

FIG. 4 Antibacterial effect of black tea fractions against cariogenic bacterium *S. mutans.*

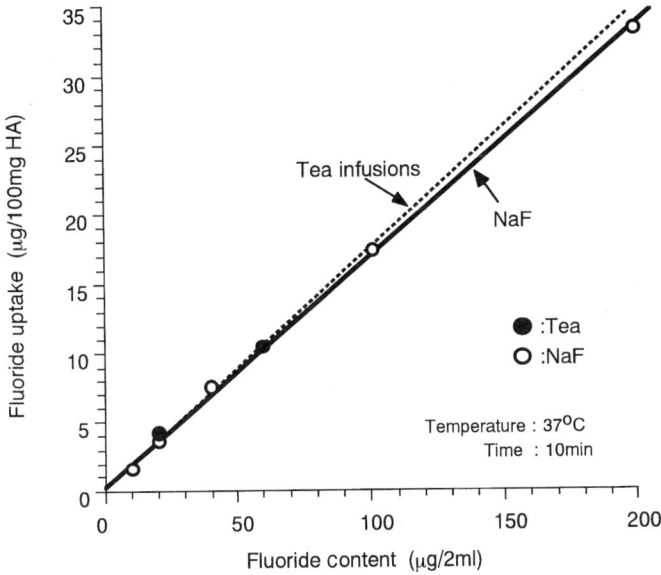

FIG. 5 Rate of fluoride uptake to HA (hydroxyapatite).

2 ml of tea extract or NaF (sodium fluoride) solution for 10 min at 37°C. As long as the concentration of fluoride in the tea solution was the same as that of the NaF solution, the rate of fluoride uptake to HA was the same, as shown in Fig. 5. This shows that fluoride absorption to the teeth will occur not only from NaF (fluoride solution), but also from tea infusion. Next, acid resistance was determined by adding 10 ml of acetate buffer (pH 4.0) and measuring the phosphate extracted into the solution from the HA. In tooth decay, the dissimilation of phosphate occurs simultaneously with that of calcium, so either phosphate or calcium may be measured to determine the acid resistancy of the solution, but analysis of the former is considerably easier.

$$\text{Acid resistancy} = \frac{\text{Amount of phosphate in the control}}{\text{Amount of phosphate in the test solution}}$$

Even though the fluoride uptake in tea solution is the same as in NaF solution, acid resistance by tea solution is

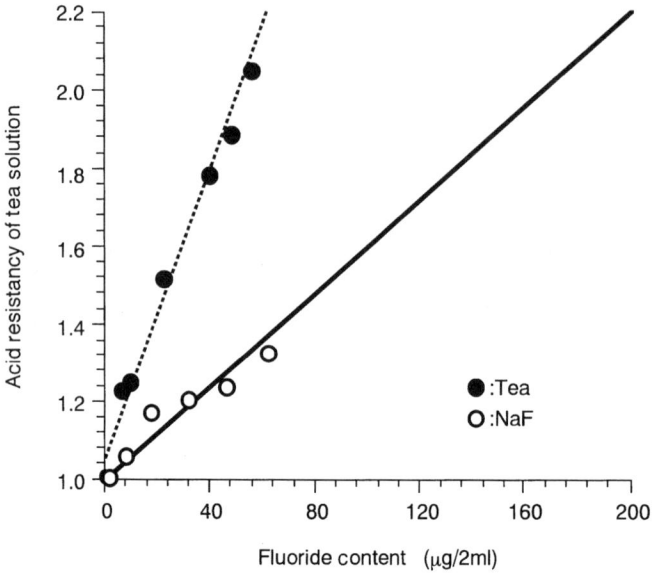

FIG. 6 Acid resistivity of hydroxyapatite treated with NaF and tea.

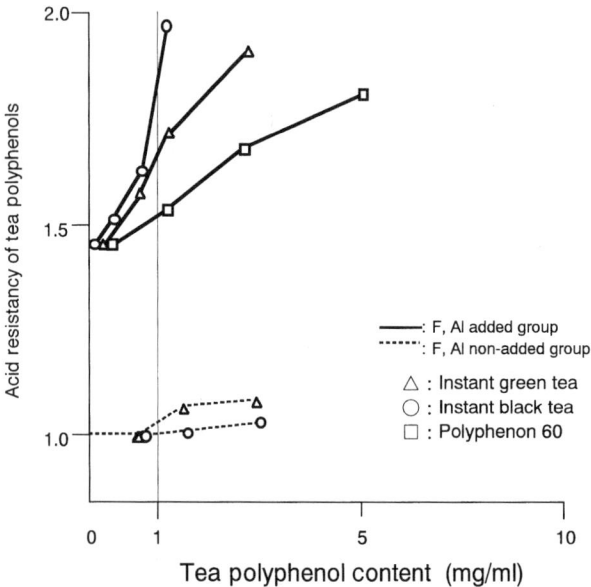

FIG. 7 Relationship between the polyphenol concentration and acid resistivity.

much stronger (Fig. 6). In the same way, aluminum ions in tea as well as polyphenolic components were found to increase the acid resistance. Conclusively, 50 µg of fluoride and 100 µg of aluminum ion was added to 2 ml of buffer solution with various amounts of tea polyphenols and acid resistancy was measured as in Fig. 7. From this graph, it could be said that the combination of tea polyphenols, fluoride, and aluminum ions (these three elements being the most abundant in tea) will increase acid resistancy of tooth enamel.

REFERENCES

1. S Kashket, VP Paolino, DA Lewis, JV Houte. In vitro inhibition of glucosyltransferase from the dental plaque bacterium *Streptococcus Mutans* by common beverages and food extracts. Archs Oral Biol 30:821–826, 1985.
2. S Sakanaka, M Kim, M Taniguchi, T Yamamoto. Antibacterial substances in Japanese green tea extract against *Streptococcus mutans*, a cariogenic bacterium. Agric Biol Chem 53:2307–2311, 1989.
3. M Onishi. The feasibility of a tea drinking program for dental public health in primary schools. J of Dental Health 35:134–143, 1985.
4. C Jin, LQ Hai, FX Zhi, LZ Zhong, JY Tao, I Oguni, Y Hara. Anticaries activity of tea: epidemiology and the role of fluorine and catechins. University of Shizuoka Junior College Research Proceedings 4:81–101, 1991.
5. M Hattori, IT Kusumoto, T Namba, T Ishigami, Y Hara. Effect of tea polyphenols on glucan synthesis by glucosyltransferase from *Streptococcus mutans*. Chem Pharm Bull 38:717–720, 1990.
6. F Hayakawa, N Kohyama, T Shiraishi, K Yoshitake, T Ando, T Kimura. The effect of green tea infusion on acid resistance of hdroxyapatite. J of Dental Health 43:48–57, 1993.

10

Antiviral Action of Tea Polyphenols

I. PLANT VIRUSES

It has been long known, especially by tobacco growers in southern Japan, that a spray containing tea extract is effective against the tobacco mosaic virus (TMV) infection. Okada investigated the active component of tea against TMV and cucumber mosaic virus (CMV) and found that tea catechins inhibit the development of these viral diseases (1). Viruses pretreated with catechins, particularly with galloyl catechins (EGCg, ECg) did not develop when applied to the leaf surface. This antiviral effect was more prominent with theaflavins. The inhibitory effect was further confirmed by administering catechins (1000 ppm and 2000 ppm) through the cut stalks of the plants for two days and then staining the leaves with the virus. When catechin solutions at 2000 ppm were administered to the roots of the tobacco plants in the soil, toxic involution appeared on the leaf edge. Catechins and theaflavins were presumed to bind to the nucleic acids of TMV and CMV and

78

inhibit their infectivity (2). While there is a strong possibility for tea polyphenols to be utilized in vegetable production, more experiments remain to be conducted to establish more practical uses.

II. INFLUENZA VIRUS

Influenza is a disease with a high mortality rate throughout the world. Despite efforts to develop effective vaccines and therapeutic agents against influenza virus infection, it is still virtually uncontrolled. The use of current vaccines against influenza virus infection is limited because of the frequent conversion of viral antigens. Symptomatic therapy is the only treatment possible for influenza virus infection except in a few countries where the antiviral compound, amantadine, is used. Although amantadine is effective in prophylaxis and therapy of the influenza A virus, it has side effects, and resistant mutants arise. Therefore, new vaccines and antiviral strategies are being explored. We recently found that tea extracts, tea polyphenols being the principal effective components, markedly inhibit infectivity of both the influenza A and B virus to MDCK (Madin-Darby canine kidney) cells by blocking their adsorption to the cells and that infection could be prevented by previous contact of the virus with tea polyphenols in animals as well as in humans.

A. Prevention of Infectivity of the Influenza Virus to the Cells (Plaque Assay)

Shimamura, Nakayama, and Hara investigated the capacity of EGCg and TF3 to inhibit infection of the influenza A and B viruses in MDCK cells (3). Influenza A/Yamagata/120/86 (NIH) and B/USSR/100/83 viruses were mixed with EGCg or TF3 either 5 min or 60 min before being exposed to the cells. MDCK cells in a six-well tissue culture plate were inoculated with the above test solutions. The control solutions (viruses alone without tea polyphenols) were appropriately diluted to grow approximately 200 pfu (plaque forming unit) viruses per plate. After allowing 60 min for virus adsorption, the cells were washed with MEM (minimum essential medium) and then overlaid with duly compounded agar. After incubation for 4 days at 33.5°C in 5% CO_2 in air, the cells were fixed with formalin, the agar overlay was removed, and the cells were stained with methylene blue. The number of plaques were counted and inhibition was calculated as against the number of plaques in the control.

As shown in Fig. 1, EGCg and TF3 almost completely inhibited infectivity of both viruses even at concentrations as

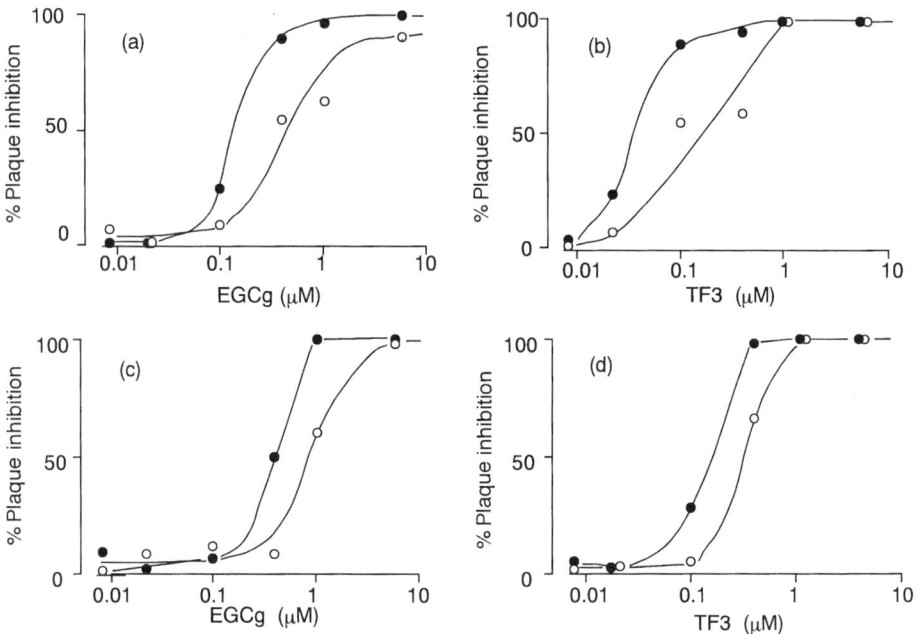

FIG. 1 Inhibitory effects of EGCg and TF3 on plaque formation by (a, b) influenza A virus and (c, d) influenza B virus. Influenza virus stocks were diluted to 2×10^3 p.f.u. ml^{-1} and incubated with various concentrations of EGCg (a, c) or TF3 (b, d) for (○) 5 min or (●) 60 min at 37°C before virus exposure to MDCK cells. The inhibition of plaque count was scored by the mean of triplicate cultures for each group after assay. Mean p.f.u. pm S.D. was 78.8 pm 22.1 of control of eight experiments.

low as 1 μM in the case of the 60 min treatment. Short-time contact (5 min) also effectively inhibited infectivity at less than 10 μM. At any rate, less than 5 ppm of EGCg or TF3 is more than enough to completely inhibit infectivity (EGCg = 458, 10 μM = 4.58 ppm). Since the concentration of tea polyphenols in an average daily cup is 500–1000 ppm, tea catechins are remarkably potent in their inhibition. Amantadine, a positive control, inhibited viral infection at a dose of approximately 50–100 times more than that of tea polyphenols in the same system.

After the viruses are adsorbed inside the cells however, tea polyphenols are only slightly effective in preventing plaque formation at more than 1000 ppm on MDCK cells. Similarly, when MDCK cells were pretreated with polyphenols and washed to remove residual polyphenols, and then challenged with the virus, plaque formation was not inhibited at concentrations of 100 μM or less.

Since the above results suggest that tea polyphenols may bind to surface glycoproteins of the influenza virus, we compared electromicroscopically the capacities of EGCg, TF3 and the anti-A virus antibody to bind to the A virus. EGCg and TF3 each at 1mM agglutinated virus particles as well as the antibody by short-time contact (Fig. 2). Viruses pretreated with EGCg (1 mM) or antibody failed to bind to MDCK cells.

The results indicate that tea polyphenols can inhibit the infectivity of the influenza virus to MDCK cells by blocking its adsorption and entry into the cells, but not its multiplication inside the cells. Though the precise molecular mechanism of antiviral activity of tea polyphenols is unclear at present, their utility in preventing the infection of the flu virus would appear to be enormous since they are effective at such a low dose and their effects are, unlike the antibody, nonspecific.

B. Animal and Human Experiments

Tea polyphenols were proven to completely inhibit infectivity of influenza viruses in vitro at concentrations as low as 10 μM.

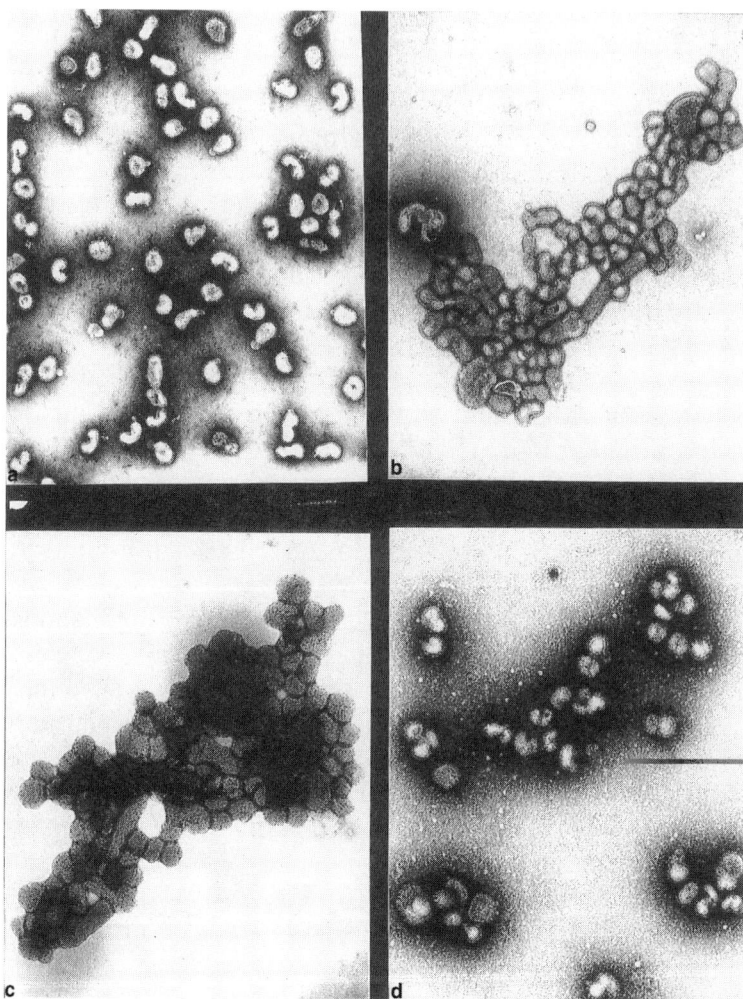

FIG. 2 Electron micrographs of influenza A virus after incubation for 5 min with (a) PBS as control, (b) 1mM EGCg, (c) 1 mM TF3, or (d) antivirus IgG (6400HI titer). Viruses were negatively stained with 2% solution phosphotung state (pH7.2).

This inhibitory action was effective through direct contact of viruses with tea polyphenols. In the following experiments we have further confirmed that once the virus is inhibited in vitro, noninfectivity will not be reversed in animals (4).

Mice infected with the influenza virus through intranasal titration (inhalation) markedly decreased in body weight and died within 10 days, whereas all mice administered viruses pretreated with tea extract achieved normal body weight increases and survivals. Three-week-old female C3H/He specific pathogen-free (SPF) mice used in this experiment were sensitive to the influenza virus A/WSN/33 (H1N1) and their i.n. LD_{50} was $10^{3.87}$ pfu/mouse. Even for inhalation of the virus at $10^{1.8}$ pfu/mouse, all mice were confirmed to be infected by detection of antibody. Black tea was extracted to a concentration of 4% (4 g/100 ml water) and mixed with the same volume of virus solution (15 ml each to make 30 ml solution) for 5 minutes. This produced 2% black tea infusion, containing viruses, to be administered to the mice. The number of viruses was adjusted to 1×10^5/mouse. The virus group was administered virus solution mixed with MEM medium in place of black tea infusion. The control group was administered MEM medium alone. The number of mice in each group was 10. As shown in Fig. 3, the body weights of the virus-MEM group began to decrease from the fourth day after inhalation and continued to further decrease over time. Fig. 4 shows abrupt deaths for the virus-MEM group after the fifth day. In this group, 50% of the mice died on the sixth day and all died by the tenth day. On the other hand, body weight gain among the virus-black tea group corresponded to weight gain in the control group (Fig. 3) and all mice survived during the test period (Fig. 4). In the virus-tea group, blood was collected from the surviving mice on the fourteenth day after inhalation and antibody production was examined. Among the 10 mice, only one showed slight antibody reaction (data not shown). This may have been caused by a few viruses remaining intact with the tea polyphenols. In any event, it is most probable that black tea of daily drinking concentration will neutralize infectivity in the

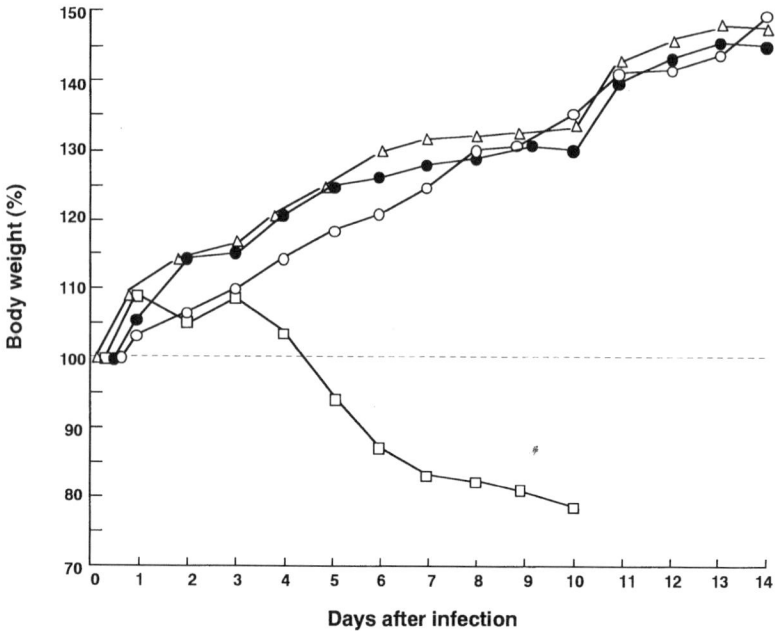

FIG. 3 Protection by tea extracts against influenza infection in mice. Mice were administered with $10^{5.3}$ p.f.u./mice ($10^{1.3}LD_{50}$) of fluvirus (WSN strain). Body weight was observed for 14 days. (○) MEM; (□) virus; (△) 2% black tea; (●) 2% black tea and virus.

influenza virus through direct contact and these effects will not be reversed even after the conjugated viruses are inhaled into the lungs. In these trials the active components in tea were confirmed as tea polyphenols.

We have conducted further antiflu experiments on pigs on a farm in northern Japan. In one pen, green tea extract powder (Polyphenon G™, catechin content 30%) was mixed with the drinking water at 0.1% concentration. At the same time, this drinking water was sprayed from a roof nozzle for 20 seconds every 30 minutes during the daytime. Blood was collected from the pigs in this pen as well as from the animals in the control group. After one month, in the control group the antibody value (measured as HI, hemagglutination inhibition)

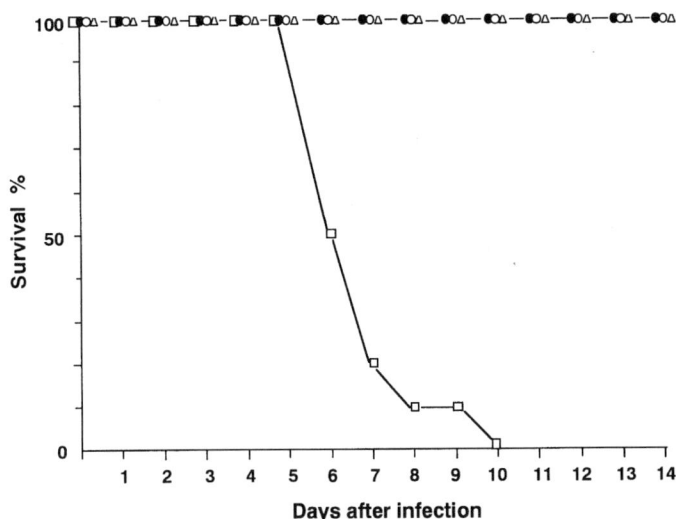

FIG. 4   Protection by tea extracts against influenza infection in mice. Mice
were administered with $10^{5.3}$ p.f.u./mice ($10^{1.3}LD_{50}$) of fluvirus (WSN strain).
Survival was observed for 14 days. (O) MEM; (□) virus; (△) 2% black tea;
(●) 2% black tea and virus.

increased more than four times, whereas in the test group the
increase of HI antibody value was significantly suppressed (5).
This indicated that there was less virus infection in the tea
group.

Human trials were also conducted where one group gar-
gled daily with canned black tea from the end of October to
the end of March while the control group did not. A significant
decrease in the number of people infected with influenza was
observed in the test group as compared to the control (6).

The above results suggest the efficacy of gargling with
tea in preventing infection during an influenza virus epidemic.
Increased preventative effects are anticipated through the use
of mouthwash, chewing gum, or drops, and these products are
already in trial, if not actual mass production, although ex-
plicit claims on the efficacy of the products has not yet been
allowed.

III. HUMAN PAPILLOMA VIRUSES

Condyloma acuminata is a wart detectable on the skin or mucous membrane of the genital organs of men and women, and is caused by human papilloma virus (HPV). This wart shows distinctive papillary or cockscomblike tumors. It has a tendency to accumulate and multiply and is usually red or reddish-brown in color. Detection of HPV in condyloma acuminata is by a method of taking tissue or a smear from the infected area and determining the DNA of the virus. According to this method the detection rate is almost 100%. Types HPV6 and 11 of the virus are the ones most commonly detected in condyloma acuminata. There are many types of papilloma viruses infecting human and animal species by the process of adsorption and entry into the host cells, where they either persist in the episomal or are integrated in the genome. Since HPV16 has been detected in malignant squamous cell carcinoma from cancer of the cervix and condyloma acuminata, there is a strong possibility that HPV16 is related to the malignancy of cervical dysplasia or condyloma acuminata. Elimination or treatment of condyloma acuminata has been conducted by surgical excisions or by applying chemicals, such as cancer drugs or those for enhancing immunity, but surgical treatment is distressing for the patient and chemical applications ensue very low compliance by the patient because of the disturbing side effects. Moreover, there is a high rate of recurrence of the warts for the treatments heretofore.

Dr. Shu-Jun Cheng of the Cancer Institute (Hospital), Beijing, the Chinese Academy of Medical Sciences, in collaboration with Mitsui Norin Co., Ltd., produced a petroleum jelly-based tea catechin ointment, which patients hospitalized in the Cancer Institute (Hospital) and diagnosed with condyloma applied themselves to the infected areas. Dosage level of tea catechins was about 12% of active catechin content (15% Polyphenon E, catechin content >80%). Seventy women applied the medication daily for two months and were examined by colposcope for evaluation. Results are shown in Table 1. Cure

TABLE 1   Effect of Tea Catechin Ointment on Genital Sites

Trial	No. of site	Cured	Improved	No effect	Response
1	9	4	3	2	78%
2	34	25	5	4	88%
3	38	17	14	7	82%
All	81	46	22	13	84%

refers to complete disappearance of the wart over the two month trial; improved refers to a >50% reduction in warts. The average rate of cured or improved of 80 warts in 70 patients was 84% (the 99.9% confidence interval is 61.2% to 90.7%). None of the patients dropped out of the trials due to difficulties from the medication, despite slight pain or inflammation of the infected area for some and itching for others. There were no moderate or serious adverse effects from application of the medication. In view of the high degree of safety of tea catechins in human exposure, and high rate of success as a cure, as well as the convenience for the patients in being able to apply themselves a treatment that causes little or no discomfort, the possibilities for this medication are great. At the time of this writing, this catechin ointment has entered the phase II tests in humans which are necessary for obtaining FDA approval for a new drug application. Efficacy for cervical intraepithelial neoplasia (CIN) and other malignancies has also been confirmed.

IV. ANIMAL VIRUSES

Many reports have investigated the antiviral effect of tea on animal viruses. John et al. showed inhibition of the proliferation of the herpes virus by a tea extract solution (7). The infectivity of the rotavirus (which causes diarrhea in infants and young children) was found to be weakened by a green tea/methanol extract (Hatta et al.) (8), while Mukoyama et al. showed the antiviral effects of epigallocatechin gallate (EGCg) and theaflavin digallate (TF3) on cultured rhesus monkey kidney

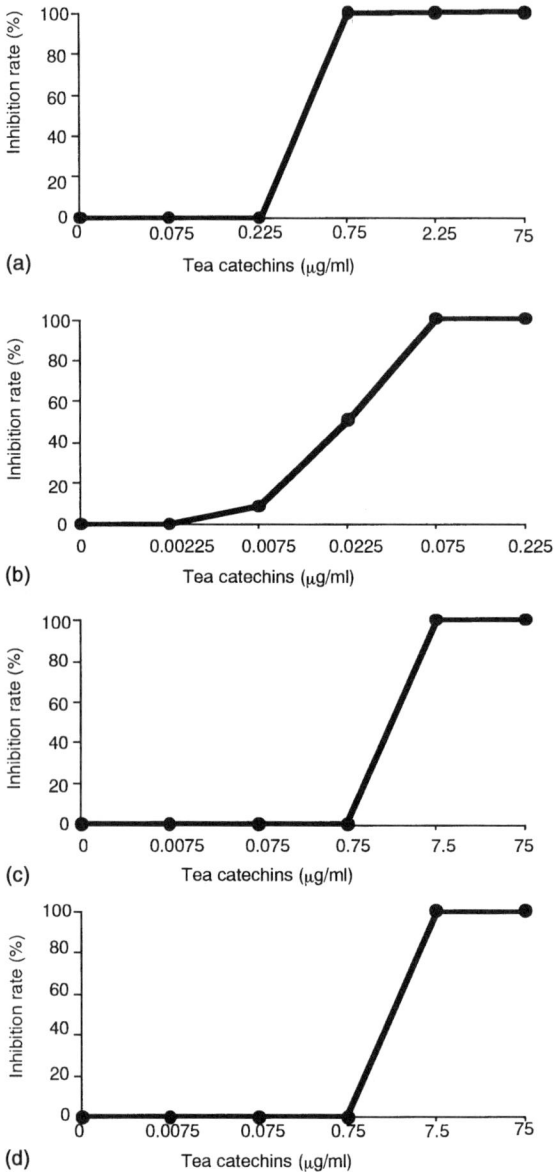

FIG. 5 Inhibitory effects of tea catechins (Polyphenon 70S) against animal viruses. (a) Aujeszky's disease virus (Pseudorabies virus); (b) bovine herpes virus 1; (c) porcine transmissible gastroenteritis virus; (d) porcine epidemic diarrhea virus.

MA 104 cells infected with rotaviruses and enteroviruses (9). In Mukoyama's study maximum effects were obtained when EGCg and TF3 were added directly to the virus while pre- and post-treatment of the cells showed a much weaker effect.

We have recently confirmed that tea catechins at concentrations less than 10 µg/ml could inactivate several viruses that cause serious epidemics in animal farming. Aujeszky's disease, caused by pseudorabies virus, is a deadly disease that claims the lives of pigs, cattle, sheep, dogs, and cats. Since grown pigs have a certain tolerance against this infection, they become carriers and spread the virus. Piglets are fatal victims. This disease is dreaded in pig farming. The vaccination apparently suppresses the disease but can not block infection. Bovine rhinotracheitis, caused by bovine herpes virus 1, makes the respiration of cattle difficult. The vaccination suppresses the disease but can not eliminate the virus. Transmissible gastroenteritis of epidemic diarrhea of pigs is caused by porcine transmissible gastroenteritis virus or porcine epidemic diarrhea virus, respectively, and young pigs often succumb to death after suffering diarrhea and vomiting. The vaccination for both of these viruses is thought to be virtually ineffective.

Solutions of viruses and tea catechins (Polyphenon 70S™, catechin content >70%) were mixed for 30 min and these samples were infected respectively on cultured cells in petri dishes. After incubating the petri dishes for 5–7 days at 37°C, the infection was observed under a microscope. As a result, as shown in Fig. 5, tea catechins (Polyphenon 70S) were confirmed to have inhibited the infection of all the above viruses at less than 10 µg/ml (10 ppm). This effective concentration of catechin is similar to that against the influenza virus. Practical applications are awaited in animal farming, with procedures for filing a patent now underway.

REFERENCES

1. F Okada. Inhibitory effects of tea catechins on the multiplication of plant virus [in Japanese]. Ann Phytopath Soc Japan 37:29–33, 1971.

2. F Okada, T Takeo, S Okada, O Takemasa. Antiviral effect of theaflavins on tobacco mosaic virus. Agric Biol Chem 41:791–794, 1977.
3. M Nakayama, K Suzuki, M Toda, S Okubo, Y Hara, T Shimamura. Inhibition of the infectivity of influenza virus by tea polyphenols. Antiviral Res 21:289–299, 1993.
4. M Nakayama, M Toda, S Okubo, Y Hara, T Shimamura. Inhibition of the infectivity of influenza virus by black tea extract [in Japanese]. The Journal of the Japanese Association for Infectious Diseases 68:824-829, 1994.
5. M Nakayama, H Ichikawa, M Toda, S Okubo, M Iwata, Y Hara, T Shimamura. Inhibition of natural infection of flu-virus on pigs by tea catechins [in Japanese]. Japanese J Bacteriol 48:323, 1993.
6. M Iwata, M Toda, T Shimamura, M Nakayama, H Tsujiyama, W Endo, O Takahashi, Y Hara, T Shimamura. Prophylactic effect of black tea extract as gargle against influenza [in Japanese]. The Journal of the Japanese Association for Infectious Diseases 71:487-494, 1997.
7. TJ John, P Mukundan. Virus inhibition by tea, caffeine and tannic acid. Indian J Med Res 69:542–545, 1979.
8. H Hatta, S Sakanaka, K Tsuda, M Kim, T Yamamoto. Antirotavirus agent in green tea [in Japanese]. Abstract of 37th Annual Meeting of Japanese Society of Virologists, Osaka, Japan, 1989, pp 327.
9. A Mukoyama, H Ushijima, S Nishimura, H Koike, M Toda, Y Hara, T Shimamura. Inhibition of rotavirus and enterovirus infections by tea extracts. Jpn J Med Sci Biol 44:181–186, 1991.

11

Prevention of Cancer by
Tea Polyphenols

I. INTRODUCTION

There is a saying that prevention is better than cure. This way of thinking certainly seems to be increasingly prevalent with regards to research into cancer. Exploding expenses for cancer therapy in the national budget will force many people involved in cancer treatment and research to explore cancer prevention methods through diet rather than concentrating on hospital cures for cancer. Cancer originates from mutagenesis brought about by various physical, chemical, and biological causes in the DNA of the cell.

Tea polyphenols have a strong radical scavenging and reducing action. They scavenge radicals produced endogenously as oxygen radicals or by exposure to radiation or UV light, as well as those produced by cancer promoters, and render them harmless; while in the digestive tract they reduce nitrite, thus preventing production of nitroso-amine, which causes cancer. Tea polyphenols also show a tendency to form strong bonds with proteins, and it is known that at low concentrations they inactivate some enzymes and viruses. There is the possibility that tea polyphenols will inactivate some viruses that cause cancer. Thus, tea polyphenols have the potential to work in a preventative way against many of the causes of cancer.

II. ANTIMUTAGENIC ACTION

Inhibitors of mutagenesis have been classified as "desmutagens" and "bioantimutagens" by Kada (1). Desmutagens are substances that directly act on mutagens chemically, enzymatically, or physically to inhibit mutagenesis, and bioantimutagens work on cells that have undergone mutagenesis to inhibit their mutagenic expression. Antimutagenic and anticarcinogenic activity of tea polyphenols are reported in various papers (2). Kada et al. have searched for bioantimutagens in natural elements as well as in foodstuffs and found bioantimutagenic activity in tea extract solution. The active component was found to be (−)-epigallocatechin gallate (EGCg) (3).

For the screening studies, the strain NIG1125 of *Bacillus subtilis* (*met his mut-1*), which has a temperature-sensitive mutation in the structural gene of DNA-polymerase III, was used. Because of this characteristic, cellular growth is stopped by elevating the temperature to 43°C. However, at 30°C, a normal rate of growth takes place with highly frequent spontaneous reverse mutations at *his* and *met* loci. Agents that lower these frequent mutations without affecting cellular growth can be considered to be bioantimutagens working at the level of DNA replication.

An overnight culture of NIG1125 in broth at 30°C was kept in an ice water mixture before use. 0.1 ml of the culture was spread on MB agar containing methionine (20 µg/ml). A paper disk impregnated with a test sample was placed at the center of the surface and the culture was incubated at 30°C for 3 days. A sample reducing the number of revertant colonies, without affecting the background growth of auxotrophic cells surrounding the disk, was considered to contain a bioantimutagen. Antibiotics producing certain growth inhibition zones without allowing spontaneous mutabilities were considered to be negative.

As a result of the above mutagenecity assay, it was found that only EGCg gave a positive result among the catechins. As shown in Fig. 1, in both histidine deficient or methionine deficient medium, EGCg dose dependently suppressed the growth of his^- → his^+ (from histidine requirement to nonhistidine requirement mutability) or met^- → met^+ at concentrations that did not affect the growth of normal cells (which require these essential amino acids). Thus, EGCg that lowers the frequency of spontaneous mutagenesis is considered to work, possibly on polymerase III, in increasing the fidelity of DNA replication. The same effect was confirmed with theaflavins which represent black tea polyphenols, though the

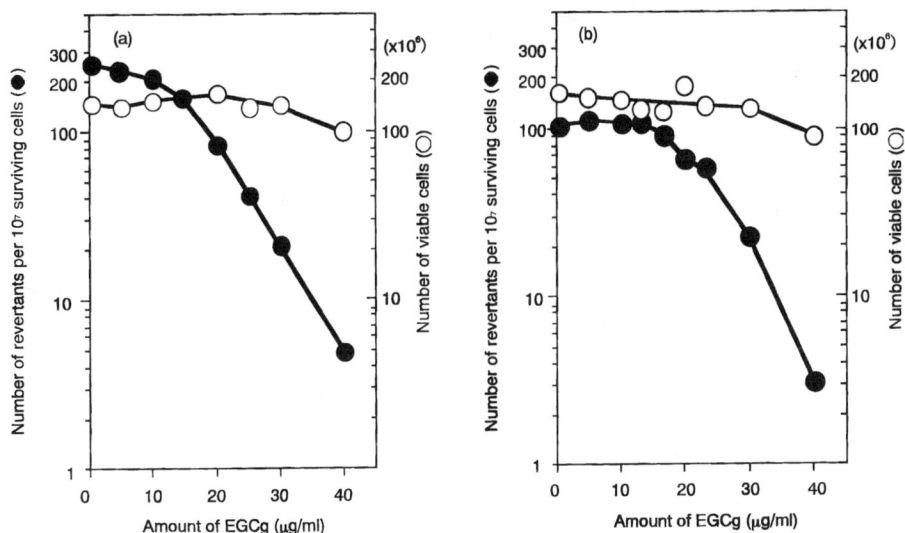

FIG. 1 Effect of EGCg on the survival and mutability in the strain *B. subtilis* NIG1125 (*his met*). (a) Reversions his^- → his^+ (b) Reversions met^- → met^+; $\bigcirc$ survivals, $\bullet$ mutations.

amount of them in black tea is only 1–2% (dry weight basis). Fig. 2 shows this effect in the case of TF3 (theaflavin digallate).

Separately, catechins with pyrogallol moiety (EGC, ECg, EGCg) showed bioantimutagenic action against UV light-induced mutagenesis in *E. coli* B/r WP2 strain which is DNA excision-repair proficient (4). This bioantimutagenic effect was not observed in the DNA excision-repair deficient strains of WP2s or ZA159.

In recent years, molecular level studies are under way on the mutagenicity of DNA in relation to oxygen radicals. Furukawa et al. reported that oxy radicals cause hydroxylation or methylation in DNA (5) and that tea catechins inhibit these sequential events. Detailed studies are awaited.

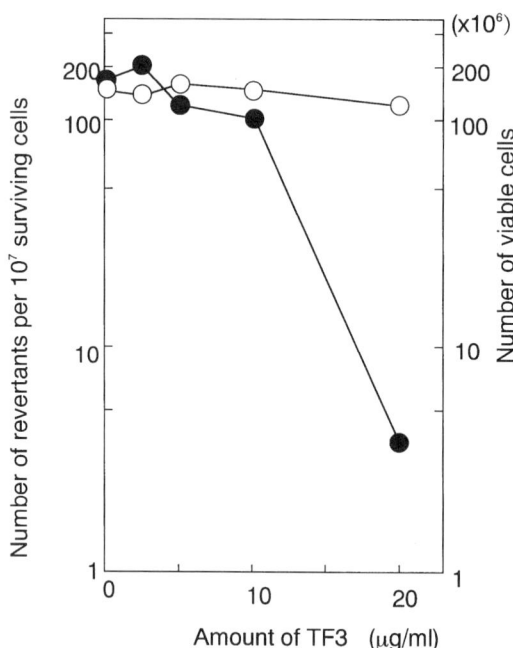

FIG. 2   Effects of TF3 on survival and mutability in the strain *B. subtilis* NIG1125 (*his met*); ○ survivals, ● mutations.

III. INHIBITION OF CHROMOSOME ABERRATIONS IN ANIMALS

The effect of EGCg on chemically-induced chromosome aberrations was investigated in vivo. Mice injected intraperitoneally with mitomycin C (MMC), as a carcinogen, developed mutations on the stem cells (erythroblast) in the femur bone marrow, and the number of erythrocytes with micronucleus fragments among the polychromatic erythrocytes (PCE) increased dose-dependently with the MMC concentration. Chemicals that reduce the above frequency are considered to work against chromosome aberrations.

EGCg (100–500 mg/kg) was administered orally to mice and 24 hours later each group was administered intraperitoneally with 2 mg/kg MMC. Another 24 hours later the bone marrow cells were taken from the mouse femur and the polychromatic erythrocytes (PCE) cells were counted. As shown in Fig. 3, the frequency of erythrocytes with micronucleus in the groups administered only MMC was 2.5% in the 1 mg/kg group, and 5.4% in the 2 mg/kg group confirming the dose de-

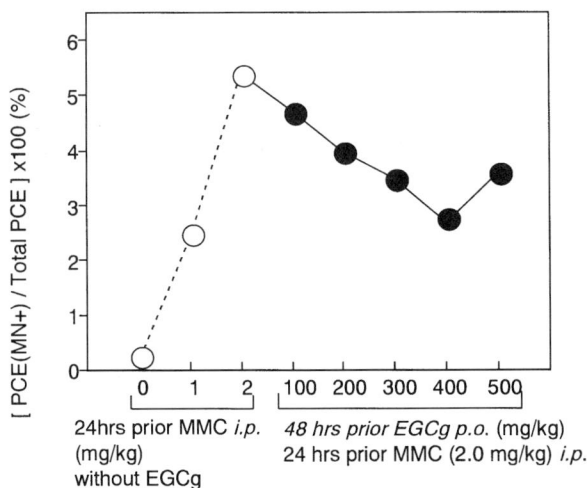

FIG. 3 Suppression of MMC-induced micronuclei by EGCg.

pendency of MMC administration on chromosome aberrations and damage to DNA (the frequency of the control without MMC was only 0.4%).

In the groups administered EGCg prior to administration of 2 mg/kg MMC, the frequency of micronuclei decreased dose dependently with the amount of EGCg administered, and at 400 mg/kg it decreased to 2.7%. Toxicity of EGCg was apparent at 500 mg/kg and there was an increase in the frequency of micronucleus fragments. These results indicate the possibility that oral administration of EGCg will inhibit chromosome aberrations.

Ito et al. investigated chromosome aberrations in rat femur bone marrow cells due to intraperitoneal administration of aflatoxin B_1 (AfB_1) and found that the frequency of chromosome aberrations was at its peak 18 hours after administration of AfB_1 (6). However, inhibition was apparent when tea catechins were administered orally to rats prior to administration of AfB_1. In particular, the most notable inhibition occurred when administration of tea catechins (450 mg/kg) was conducted 24 hours before administration of AfB_1.

MMC is a mutagen that acts directly on DNA, and AfB_1 gains mutagenicity after undergoing metabolic activation in the liver. From the above results, it is inferred that tea catechins work not only on the metabolic process of the mutagen (in the case of AFB$_1$) but they might also work on the repairing process of the mutated cells and reduce chromosome aberrations (in the case of MMC). In both cases, the fact that catechin administration was most effective 24 hours before and noneffective less than 2 hours before the injection of the carcinogen is noteworthy. For catechins, it seems that the time for absorption, distribution and/or metabolic changes in the body might be crucial in these anticarcinogen actions.

IV. ANTIPROMOTION ACTION

When a promoter acts repeatedly on a living organism whose DNA has been mutated by an initiator, cancer is induced. If

repeated administrations of a substance before and after administration of the promoter inhibit cancer in the body then
that substance can be said to have an antipromotion action.
Components of tea, particularly EGCg, have been proven to
have an antipromotion action. Fujiki et al. applied an initiator
(DMBA) to the backs of mice and then twice a week for 25
weeks a promoter, teleocidin, was applied (7). In the test group
5 mg EGCg was applied 15 minutes before each application
of teleocidin. Results showed that as compared with the control, the number of tumors in the test group was markedly
less. They also confirmed the effectiveness of EGCg using another promoter, okadaic acid, which has a different mechanism than teleocidin (8). It was hypothesized that EGCg has
a "sealing effect," that is, EGCg seals the promoter receptors
on the cells and prevents the binding of the promoter to the
cells.

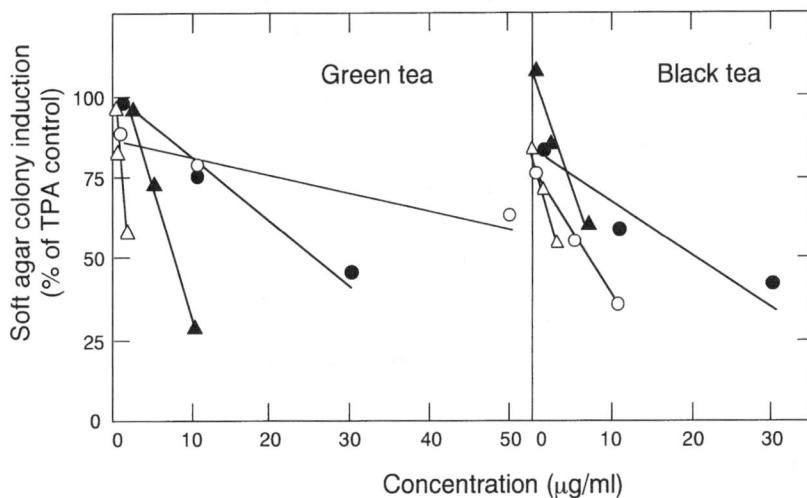

FIG. 4 Inhibition of TPA-induced neoplastic transformation (JB6 cells).
●: Chloroform fraction; △: Ethylacetate fraction; ▲: Buthanol fraction;
○: Aqueous fraction. (From Ref. 9.)

Nakamura et al. conducted experiments using JB6 cultured cells from the epidermis of Balb/C mice (9). These cells have already genetically undergone an initiation process and only with the action of a promoter (TPA) do malignant transformations occur and colonies form. The number of colonies on plates treated with components of tea at the same time as TPA decreased dose-dependently with an increasing concentration of tea (Fig. 4). It is confirmed separately that this is due not to the interaction of tea components and TPA , nor to the inhibition of the growth of transformed cells, but to the action of tea components on the promotion process by TPA. Nakamura confirmed this action with other polyphenolic complexes in tea besides EGCg and theaflavins.

V. ANTITUMOR ACTIONS IN ANIMALS

As we have seen, there is evidence that tea polyphenols work in vitro to prevent carcinogenesis. Further, the antitumor effect of tea polyphenols was investigated in the following experiments: in animals inoculated with tumor cells, in those administered a carcinogen, and in those that develop tumors spontaneously. Tea catechins (GTC, extracted from green tea, 90% purity) and a complex of tea catechins with aluminum was used (catechins were complexed with aluminum hydrochloride to reduce pungency; the complex is confirmed to separate catechins in the stomach).

First, the inhibition of the growth of inoculated cells by tea catechin was investigated. When tumor cells were injected intraperitoneally to mice, the growth of the cells in the abdominal liquid (ascites) was so rapid and vigorous that administration of tea catechins by any concentration or by any route was hardly effective in extending survival time much longer than the control. However, when tumor cells (about 10^6 cells from ascites tumors) or a tiny chip of the tumor from another mouse was implanted into the skin of mice and tea catechins were administered orally or intraperitoneally, a notable inhibition of tumor growth was observed.

In one example, mice were divided into 3 groups: the control and two groups administered catechin 0.5% and 1.0%, respectively, in their feed. Catechins were fed for a period of nine months and then tumor cells (sarcoma 180) were implanted subcutaneously around the loin. Nineteen days later, tumors from mice in all groups were weighed. As shown in Fig. 5, in the 1% catechin group the tumor weight was less than half that of the control. Separately, we have confirmed that without prior feeding of catechins similar tumor suppressive effects are obtainable if only due amount of catechins are loaded to mice. In a second example, the carcinogen 3MC (3-methylcholanthrene) was administered subcutaneously to the loin area of mice, and a catechin-aluminum complex was added to the feed for a long period of time. Results showed that, compared with the control, the formation of tumors was delayed in the catechin fed group (Fig. 6). In a third example, the effect of catechin feeding on the occurrence of tumors in a certain

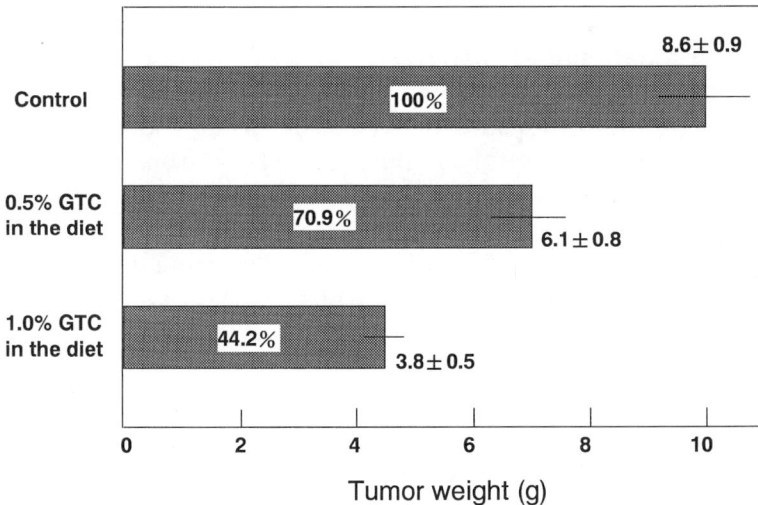

FIG. 5   Effect of GTC on Sarcoma 180 bearing ddY mice. After nine months of feeding on catechins, sarcoma cells were inoculated subcutaneously. Tumors were resected 19 days after the inoculation of tumor cells.

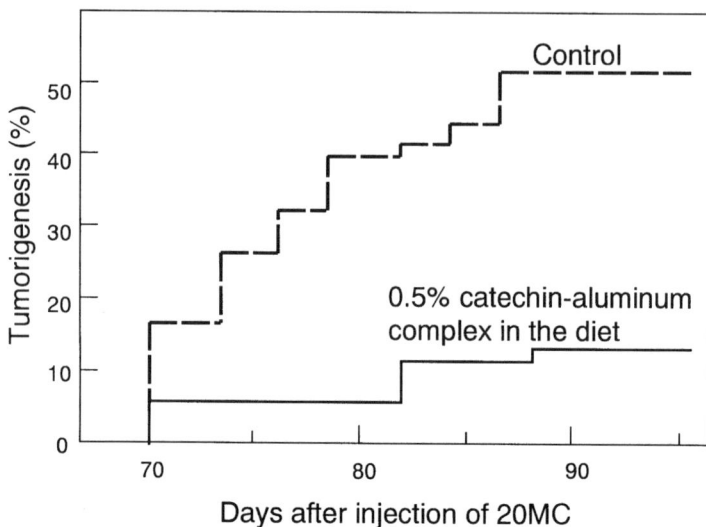

FIG. 6 Effect of catechin-aluminum complex on 3-methylcholanthrene (3MC)-induced tumorigenesis.

strain of female mice (C3H/HeN, MMTV (+)) that spontaneously develop breast cancer was investigated. As shown in Fig. 7, there was no difference between the group fed catechins (0.2% catechin-aluminum complex in the feed) from the 180th day after birth and the control group. However, in the group fed catechins from the 60th day after birth, the development of tumors was delayed. Moreover, in the offspring of mice fed catechins from birth onwards and whose mothers were fed catechins before giving birth, the development of tumors was delayed even more.

Various other experiments using different carcinogens, in different routes and in varying amounts have been conducted to study the effect of catechin administration in mice or rats and tea catechins have been proven to be effective in suppressing the development of tumors in the digestive tract, skin and various other organs (10–12).

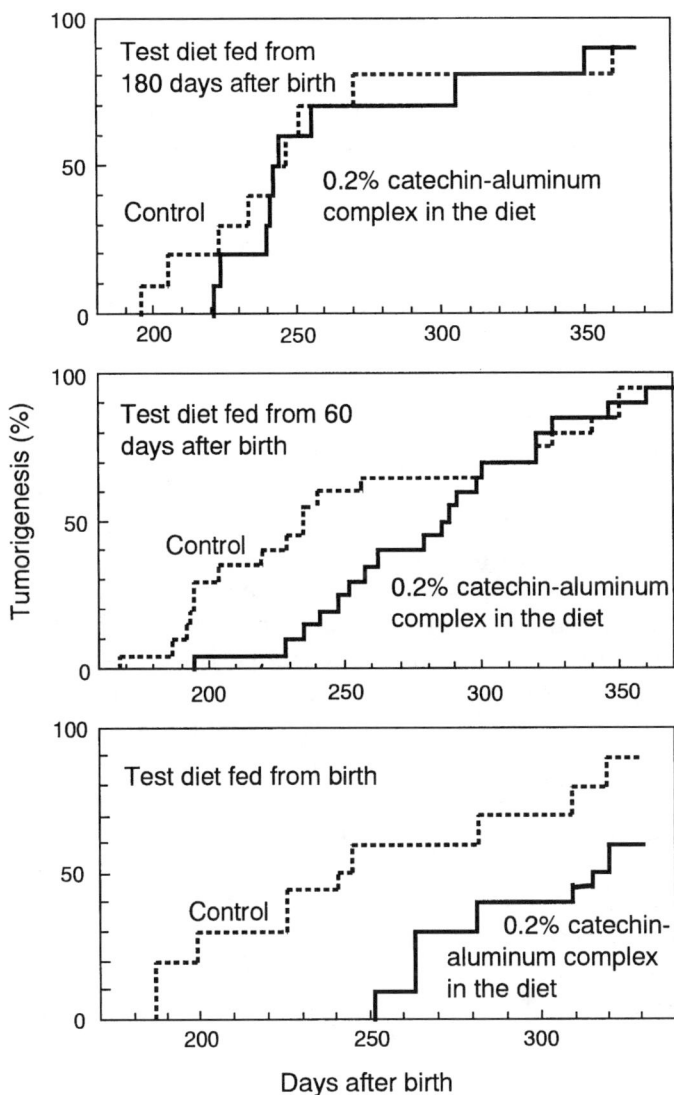

FIG. 7 Inhibition of spontaneous mammary tumor incidence in CH3/HeN strain by catechin-aluminum complex fed in the diet.

VI. EPIDEMIOLOGY

Thus, tea polyphenols have been shown to inhibit the development of tumors both in vitro and in animal experiments. Further, epidemiological studies on the influence of tea polyphenol intake (that is, tea drinking on cancer) have revealed some favorable results.

Half of the total amount of tea produced in Japan comes from Shizuoka Prefecture and it was discovered that in a certain part of that prefecture the standardized mortality rate (SMR) for stomach cancer was considerably low, i.e., 20% of the national average. That area was a high producer of tea, and it was confirmed that the residents there consumed much more tea than in nonproducing areas (13).

Another study in Japan investigated the dietary habits of three groups: patients with stomach cancer, outpatients without cancer, and nonpatients. These three groups were divided into those that drank more than five cups of tea a day, those that drank more than 10 cups a day, and those that hardly drank any. It was found that the percentage of those with cancer in the group that drank more than 10 cups a day was about half that of those in the group that hardly drank any tea at all (14).

These results indicate that by drinking lots of tea regularly, the processes that result in cancer may be prevented, thus bringing about a reduction in the incidence of stomach and other cancers. There have been many other reports on the effects of tea beverages on cancer. Based on the previous research, there has been a definite move toward investigating whether or not tea polyphenols prevent cancer in humans through intervention trials (15).

A. *Helicobacter pylori*

Recently, the bacterium *Helicobacter pylori* has come to be regarded as a possible cause of stomach cancer. It is thought that this bacterium grows in the mucous membrane of the stomach, damaging the membrane and causing peptic ulcers, which may ultimately develop into cancer of the stomach. This bacterium metabolizes urea and produces ammonia which neutralizes surrounding acidity in the stomach and enables the survival of the bacterium. Antibiotics that act to destroy the bacteria could prevent the development of ulcers and possibly stomach cancer. Yet, the use of antibiotics could be avoided if there is an element in natural foodstuffs that would work in the same way. Tea catechins have a strong antibacterial action against *H. pylori* at a concentration even half or less of that contained in ordinary tea brew as shown in Table 1. Thus, human intervention trials are under way to investigate whether the administration of tea polyphenols could eliminate *H. pylori*. In 1996, 34 people who were confirmed carriers of *H. pylori* in Hamamatsu Medical Center in Shizuoka Prefecture took seven capsules of catechins a day (one capsule contained 100 mg catechins, i.e., one to two tea cups worth) for a period of one month (16). For the determination of *H. pylori*, ^{13}C Urea was given to the subject and the metabolized $^{13}CO_2$ (by the bacterium) was measured. With a decrease in the number of the bacteria, the labeled carbon dioxide count would decrease. The results in Fig. 8 show the decrease of ^{13}C count in most of the subjects. Among the subjects, six people seemed to be free from *H. pylori*, with a

TABLE 1   Minimum Inhibitory Concentration (MIC) of Catechins for Standard Strains and Clinical Isolates of *H. pylori* (μg/ml)

	EGCg	ECg	EGC	EC
ATCC 43526	50	50	200	>200
ATCC 43629	50	50	>200	>200
ATCC 43579	50	50	200	>200
CAM(−) (n = 8)	50[a]	50[a]	200[a]	200[a]
CAM(+) (n = 12)	50[a]	50[a]	200[a]	>200[a]

Abb: ATCC, American type culture collection (standard strain); CAM(−), clarithromycin resistant strain; CAM(+), clarithromycin sensitive strain; EC, Epigallocatechin; EGC, Epigallocatechin; ECg, Epigallocatechin gallate; EGCg, Epigallocatechin gallate.

[a] MIC_{50} values were expressed.

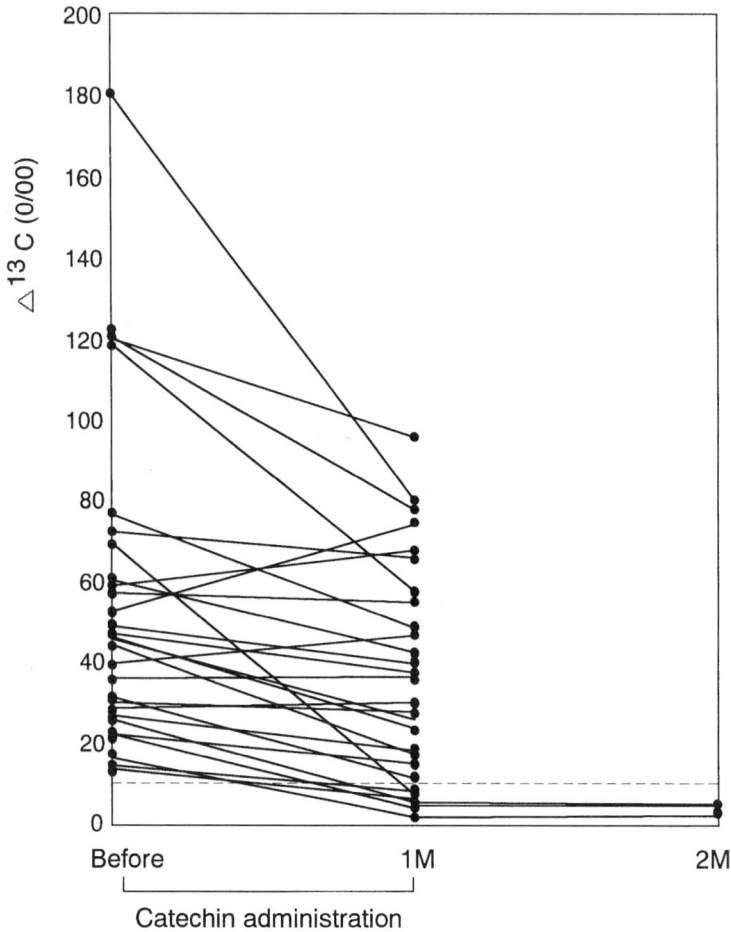

FIG. 8 Changes in ^{13}C-urea breath (^{13}CO$_2$) before, 1 month after catechin intake (1M), and 1 month after termination of catechin intake (2M).

count of less than 1% of labeled carbon. One month later, after the finish of the catechin intake, the elimination of the bacterium was confirmed with those six subjects. The counts of the rest of the people increased again showing the growth of the bacteria had resumed after termination of catechin administration.

VII. INDUCTION OF APOPTOSIS AND PREVENTION OF INVASION AND METASTASIS

Apoptosis is programmed cell death, as opposed to necrosis, which is accidental cell death. In necrosis, damaged cells or the tissues thereof undergoes bloating, rupture, and inflammation as seen in cuts or bruises. In apoptosis, cells tend to at first shrink in size followed by fragmentation of DNA; then the cell breaks into small pieces, i.e., apoptotic bodies, which are absorbed or eaten by the neighboring normal cells or by leucocytes. Examples of programmed cell death (apoptosis) are the disappearance of a tail from tadpole or webs from the fetal hands of a human baby. It would be most desirable if apoptosis could be induced specifically on the cancer cells without damaging normal cells. Several chemotherapeutic drugs are known to have apoptosis-inducing potency, but these also have side effects on normal cells.

Hibasami et al. found that tea catechins as well as the polyphenolic fraction of persimmon extract induce apoptosis in human lymphoid leukemia cells (Molt 4B), dose and time dependently (17). Furthermore, Hara and Hibasami have confirmed that tea catechins induce apoptosis in human stomach cancer cells, KATO III (18). Morphological changes are shown in Fig. 9. As against nontreated KATO III cells (a), 1 mM EGCg (b) and 0.5 mg/ml polyphenon 70S™ (catechin content

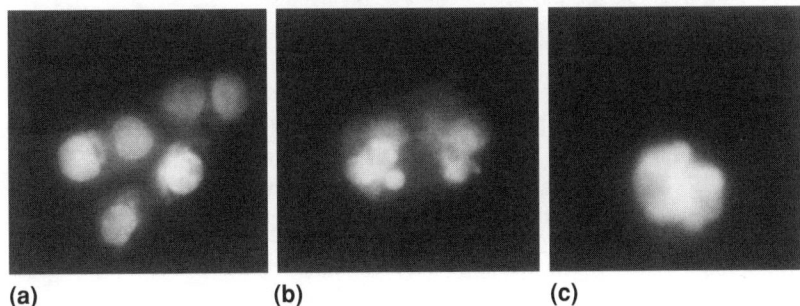

(a)   (b)   (c)

FIG. 9   Morphological changes of KATO III cells.

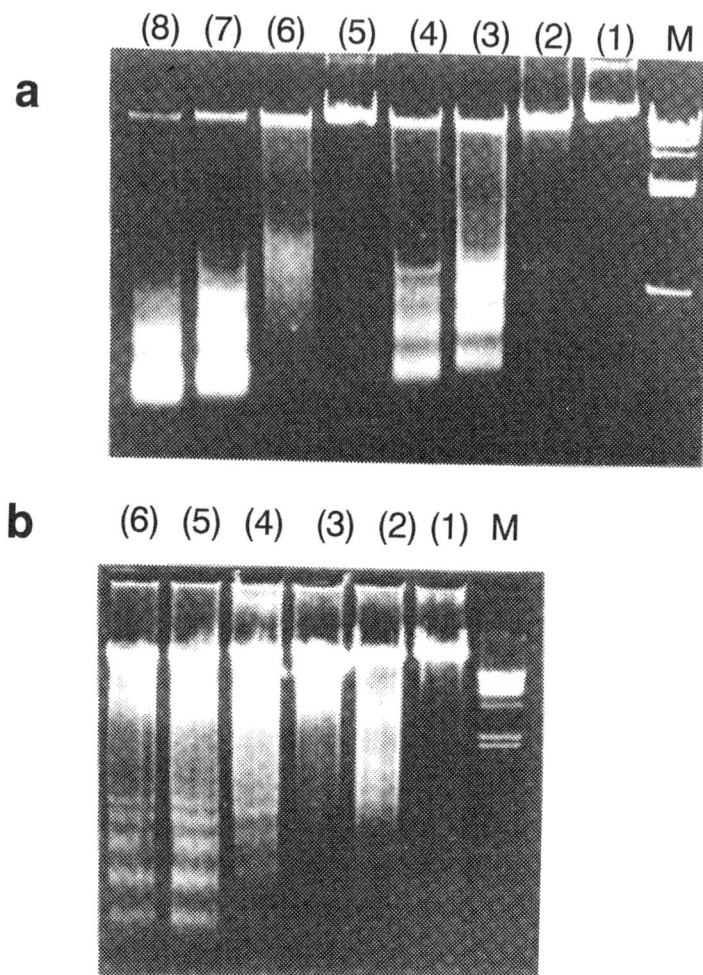

FIG. 10 (a) Time course and dose dependency of induction of apoptosis by green tea catechins. M: λ DNA digested with Hind III. (1) Control, (2) 1 day, (3) 2 days, (4) 3 days. Each treated with 0.5 mg/ml polyphnon 70S™. (5) Control, (6) 1 day, (7) 2 days, (8) 3 days. Each treated with 1 mg/ml of poly-phenon 70S™. (b) Dose dependency of apoptosis induction by EGCg. (1) Control, (2) 0.1 mM, (3) 0.2 mM, (5) 0.4 mM, (6) 1 mM. Each treated for three days.

> 70%) (c) produced apoptotic bodies in 2 days treatment. Control cells (a) lack the morphologic characteristics of an apoptotic body. The concentrations of EGCg or polyphenon 70S correspond to rather weaker than normal drinking brew (50–100 mg catechins/100 ml water is an average cup and therefore 1 mM EGCg = 45.8 mg EGCg/100 ml, 0.5 mg P-70S/1 ml = 37.5 mg catechins/100 ml). DNA fragmentation is shown in Fig. 10.

These findings suggest that polyphenons or their major component, EGCg, might exert antitumor activity in humans by triggering apoptosis and that proliferation of cancer cells may be suppressed by the presence of tea catechins. Experi-

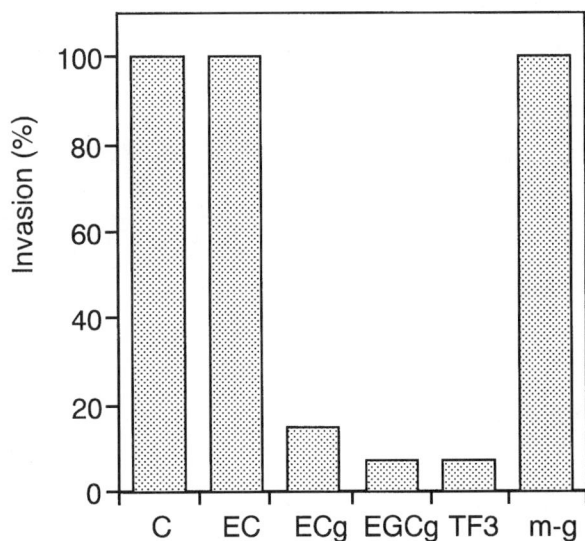

FIG. 11 Effects of tea polyphenols on matrigel invasion. Cell suspensions (100 μl) and 100 ml of green tea catechins or galloyl compounds were added to each upper compartment of the chemotaxicell chambers, and the culture medium (500 μl) containing each test sample was added to each well of the microplate. Final concentrations were 100 μM. After incubation (37°C, 6–8 h), the upper surface of the filters were wiped away and the number of control was taken as 100%. m-g, methyl gallate.

ments with other human cancer cells as well as with black tea
polyphenols are in progress.

One of the most dreadful facts about cancer is its metastatic nature. If there were no metastasis, cancer could be
manageable. Isemura et al. inoculated highly metastatic
mouse Lewis lung carcinoma cells, LL2-Lu3 (1×10^6), subcutaneously into mice (19,20). Thereafter, either green tea infusion (2 g/100 ml) or tap water was given to the group of mice
ad libitum. After three weeks, the weight and number of tumors in the lung were counted. Results showed that the number of tumors developed in the lung of the tea group was almost half that of the control group, demonstrating in vivo the
antimetastatic effect of tea infusion. In vitro experiments revealed that galloyl catechins (EGCg, ECg) and theaflavins at
a dose of 100 μM inhibit the invasion of LL2-Lu3 into matrigel

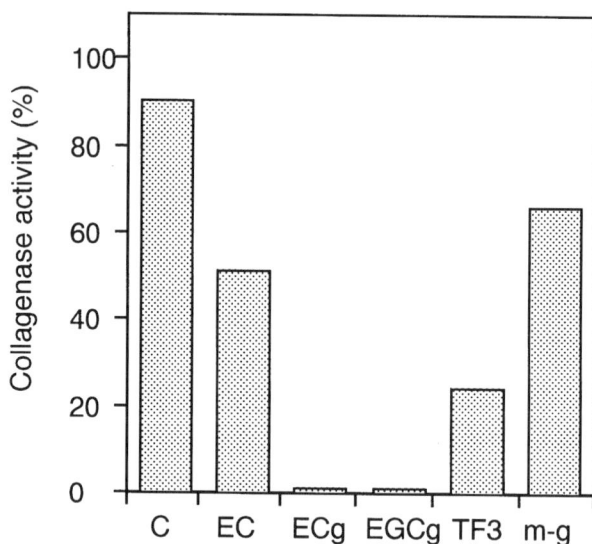

FIG. 12 Effects of tea polyphenols on type IV collagenase activity. The collagenase activity was measured in the presence or absence (control) of the
test inhibitor solution (200 μM) with fluorescein isothiocyanate-labeled type
IV collagen. The value for the control was taken as 100%. m-g, methyl gallate.

(a model of basement membrane) as shown in Fig. 11, which will eventually result in the inhibition of metastasis in the living system. Free catechins (C, EC) or methyl gallate did not show any anti-invasive effect. Isemura postulated this anti-invasive action of galloyl catechins and theaflavins to be the inhibition of enzymes produced by cancer cells in invasion and demonstrated colagenase inhibition of these catechins and theaflavins as shown in Fig. 12.

REFERENCES

1. T Kada, T Inoue, T Ohta, Y Shirasu. Antimutagens and their modes of action. In: DM Shankel, PE Hartman, T Kada, A Hollaender, ed. Antimutagenesis and Anticarcinogenesis Mechanisms. New York: Plenum Press, 1986, pp 181–196.
2. Y Kuroda, Y Hara. Antimutagenic and anticarcinogenic activity of tea polyphenols. Mut Res 436:69–97, 1999.
3. T Kada, K Kaneko, S Matsuzaki, T Matsuzaki, Y Hara. Detection and chemical identification of natural bioantimutagens— A case of the green tea factor. Mut Res 150:127–132, 1985.
4. K Shimoi, Y Nakamura, I Tomita, Y Hara, T Kada. The pyrogallol related compounds reduce UV-induced mutations in *Escherichia coli* B/r WP2. Mut Res 173:239–244, 1986.
5. H Furukawa, J Ebata, M Toyohara, N Ito, A Imoto, K Kuritki, T Hohmi, T Sofuni. Oxy-radical mechanism in mutagenicity expression of *N*-nitrosodimethylamine in ames test. Proceedings of the 2nd International Conference on Bioradicals, Yamagata, Japan, 1997, pp 57–59.
6. Y Ito, S Ohnishi, K Fujie. Chromosome aberrations induced by aflatoxin B_1 in rat bone marrow cells in vivo and their suppression by green tea. Mut Res 222:253–261, 1989.
7. S Yoshizawa, T Horiuchi, H Fujiki, T Yoshida, T Okuda, T Sugimura. Antitumor promoting activity of (−)-epigallocatechin gallate, the main constituent of "tannin" in green tea. Phytotherapy Res, 1:44–47, 1987.
8. S Yoshizawa, T Horiuchi, M Suganuma, S Nishikawa, J Yatsunami, S Okabe, T Okuda, Y Muto, K Frenkel, W Troll, H Fujiki. Pento-*O*-galloyl-β-D-glucose and (−)-epigallocatechin gallate– cancer preventive agents. In: MT Huang, CT Ho, CY Lee, ed.

Phenolic Compounds in Food and their Effects on Health II. Washington: American Chemical Society, 1992, pp 316–325.

9. Y Nakamura, S Harada, I Kawase, M Matsuda, I Tomita. Inhibitory effects of tea ingredients on the in vitro tumor promotion of mouse epidermal JB6 cells. Proceedings of the International Symposium on Tea Science. Shizuoka, Japan, 1991, pp 205–209.

10. CS Yang, ZY Wang. Review—tea and cancer. J Nat Cancer Inst 85:1038–1049, 1993.

11. S Katiyar, H Mukhtar. Tea in chemoprevention of cancer: epidemiologic and experimental studies (review). Int J Onc 8:221–238, 1996.

12. LA Mitscher, M Jung, D Shankel, JH Dou, L Steele, SP Pillai. Chemoprotection: a review of the potential therapeutic antioxidant properties of green tea (Camellia sinensis) and certain of its constituents. Med Res Rev 17:327–365, 1997.

13. I Oguni, K Nasu, S Kanaya, Y Ota, S Yamamoto, T Nomura. Epidemiological and experimental studies on the antitumor activity by green tea extracts. Jpn J Nutr 47:93–102, 1989.

14. S Kono, M Ikeda, S Tokudome, M Kuratsune. A case-control study of gastric cancer and diet in Northern Kyushu, Japan. Jpn J Cancer Res 79:1067–1074, 1988.

15. NCI, DCPC Chemoprevention Branch and Agent Development Committee. Clinical development plan: tea extracts green tea polyphenols epigallocatechin gallate. J Cellular Biochem 265:236–257, 1996.

16. M Yamada, B Murohisa, M Kitagawa, Y Takehira, K Tamakoshi, N Mizushima, T Nakamura, K Hirasawa, T Horiuchi, I Oguni, N Harada, Y Hara. Effects of tea polyphenols against Helicobacter pylori. In: T Shibamoto, J Terao, T Osawa ed. Functional Foods for Disease Prevention I, Fruits, Vegetables, and Teas. ACS Symposium Series 701: American Chemical Society, 1998, pp 217–224.

17. H Hibasami, Y Achiwa, T Fujikawa, T Komiya. Induction of programmed cell death (apoptosis) in human lymphoid leukemia cells by catechin compounds. Anticancer Res 16:1943–1946, 1996.

18. H Hibasami, T Komiya, Y Achiwa, K Ohnishi, T Kojima, K Nakanishi, K Akashi, Y Hara. Induction of apoptosis in human stomach cells by green tea catechins. Onc Rep 5:527–529, 1998.

19. M Isemura, M Sazuka, H Imazawa, T Nakayama, T Noro, Y Nakamura, Y Hara. Inhibitory effects of green tea infusion on in vitro and in vivo metastasis of mouse lung carcinoma cells. In: H Ohigashi, T Osawa, J Terao, T Yoshikawa, ed. Food Factors for Cancer Pevention, Tokyo: Springer-Verlag, 1997, pp 134–137.

20. M Sazuka, H Imazawa, Y Shoji, T Mita, Y Hara, M Isemura. Inhibition of collagenases from mouse lung carcinoma cells by green tea catechins and black tea theaflavins. Biosci Biotech Biochem 61:1504–1506, 1997.

12

Lipid Lowering Effects

I. INTRODUCTION

There is a great deal of evidence that dietary fat, dietary cholesterol, sugar, protein, and fiber can influence plasma cholesterol levels and atherogenesis in experimental animals and in humans. Relatively little attention has been paid to polyphenols and tannins in foodstuffs. Würsch reported a reduction in plasma cholesterol in rats fed polymerized tannins (1). Okuda et al. observed that tea tannins inhibit the elevation of serum cholesterol levels when administered to rats fed a peroxidized corn oil diet (2). Fukuo et al. reported that the blood total cholesterol levels in human subjects, who habitually drank a mixture of three egg yolks in dense green tea brew every day for 21 years, were within the normal range and suggested that tannins (i.e., catechins) in green tea may be involved in the maintenance of normal blood cholesterol levels (3).

II. SHORT TERM HIGH-FAT DIET

In this study, the effects of tea catechins on lipid metabolism were investigated in male weanling rats fed a cholesterol elevating high-fat diet for 28 days (4). As shown in Table 1, the high-fat diet was composed of, in addition to 25% casein: 15% lard, 15% sucrose, and 1% cholesterol which took the place of some of the α-starch component. Green tea catechin (GTC) was supplemented at 1% of this high-fat diet. The high-fat diet increased plasma LDL cholesterol, liver lipids, and liver cholesterol markedly and tended to decrease plasma HDL cholesterol as compared to the control group. Fig. 1 shows the remarkable increase of LDL cholesterol by the high-fat diet and the suppression of it with the addition of 1% GTC. The reduction of HDL cholesterol by the high-fat diet tended to be rectified by GTC. In the same way, the marked increase of liver fats was suppressed by GTC as shown in Fig. 2. On the contrary, tea catechin supplementation in-

TABLE 1   Composition of Diets (%)

Ingredients	25C[a]	25CLC	25CLC + 1% GTC
Casein	25.0	25.0	25.0
Corn oil	5.0	2.0	2.0
Lard	—	15.0	15.0
Sucrose	—	15.0	15.0
α-corn starch	63.9	35.8	34.9
Vitamin mixture[b]	1.0	1.0	1.0
Salt mixture[b]	5.0	5.0	5.0
Choline chloride	0.1	0.1	0.1
Cholesterol	—	1.0	1.0
GTC	—	—	1.0

The diets also contained retinyl acetate (2,000IU), ergocalciferol (2001U) and α-tocopherol (0.01g) per 100g of diet.
[a] 25C; (25% casein), 25CLC; (25C + 15% lard + 1% cholesterol), 25CLC + 1% GTC; (25CLC + 1% GTC).
[b] From Harper, A.E. (1959): J. Nutr., 68, 405.

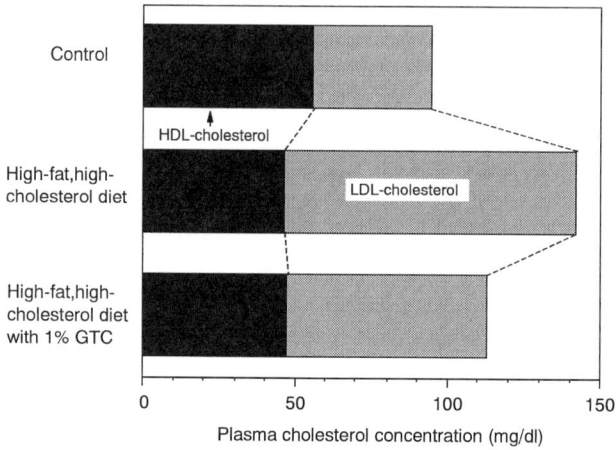

FIG. 1 Hypocholesterolemic effect of GTC in rats fed a high-fat and high-cholesterol diet.

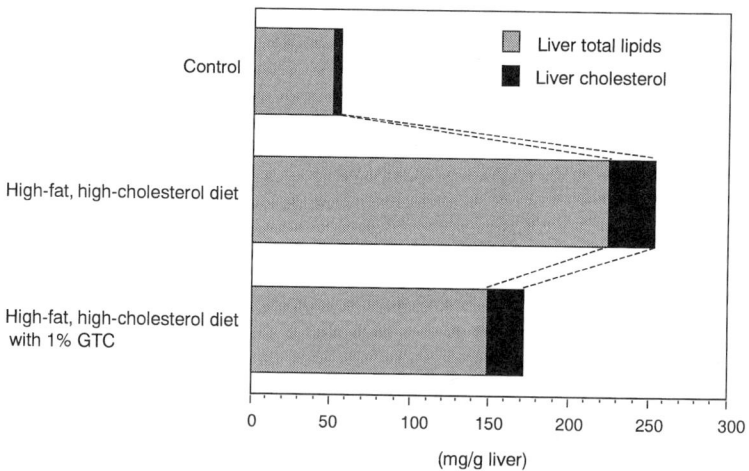

FIG. 2 Effect of GTC on liver lipid concentrations in rats fed a high-fat and high-cholesterol diet.

creased fecal excretion of total lipids and cholesterol as shown in Fig. 3.

More pronounced results were obtained in experiments where 0.5% and 1% of EGCg were added to the high-fat diet (5). Fig. 4 shows a phenomenal increase of plasma LDL cholesterol by the high-fat diet and a marked suppression of it by EGCg. The reduction of liver fats and the increase of excreted fats were more prominently demonstrated than in the previous experiment.

The results demonstrate that tea catechins exert a hypocholesterolemic effect in rats fed high-fat/sucrose/cholesterol diet. Moreover, tea catechins were shown to arrest the decrease of an essential factor, i.e., plasma HDL cholesterol. As one of the mechanisms of these functions of tea catechins, Sugano et al. reported the fact that dietary catechins, particularly galloyl catechins (EGCg and ECg) will reduce the solubility of cholesterol in mixed micelles, thus reducing the absorption of cholesterol from the intestine (6). Quite interestingly, we have confirmed that when 1% of EGCg is mixed in the normal diet and not in the high-fat diet, none

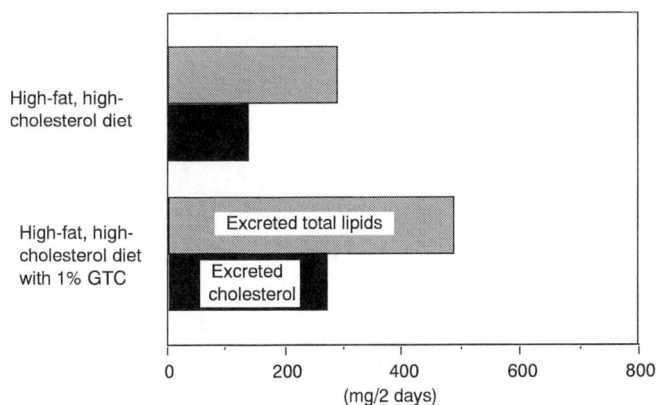

FIG. 3 Effect of GTC on fecal excretion of total lipids and cholesterol in rats fed a high-fat and high-cholesterol diet.

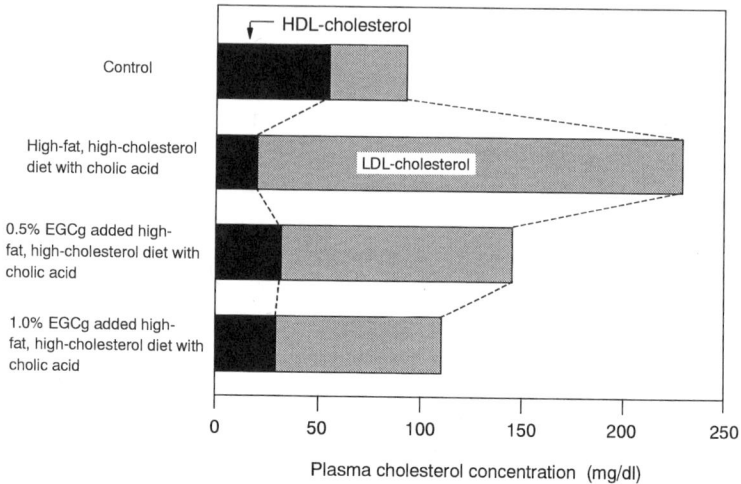

FIG. 4 Hypocholesterolemic effect EGCg in rats fed a high-fat and high-cholesterol diet with cholic acid.

of the parameters such as content of plasma cholesterol and liver fats, or body weight and food intake showed any significant differences between the control and EGCg groups during the seven weeks of this diet being consumed (5). Differences were noted in increased total lipids and cholesterol in the feces and the doubled bulk of the feces by EGCg feeding. These facts suggest that no malnutrition by catechin intake will occur, but that only in the case when extra fats and sucrose are taken catechins will work to prevent the impending health disorders that may be caused by excess nutrients. Similar results were obtained by administering 1% black tea polyphenols (BTP, mainly composed of thearubigin fraction) in the high-fat, high-cholesterol diet. Significant reduction of total cholesterol, phospholipid and triglyceride concentrations in plasma was observed in less than a month feeding (7). These results indicated that certain amount of tea polyphenols in the diet might be effective in ameliorating hyperlipidemia.

III. LIFELONG NORMAL DIET

In yet another animal experiment, we confirmed the merit of catechin intake on a lifelong basis (8). The supplementation of green tea catechin (GTC) in the normal diet (0.5% and 1.0%) of rats was performed from weanling (three weeks of age) to 19 months old (rats live a little longer than two years). A significant suppression of body weight gain by tea was observed only at 7–11 weeks of age, but there were no significant changes in liver and kidney weight between the control group and GTC fed groups. Noticeable are the contents of plasma lipids (triglyceride (TG), total cholesterol (TC), and phospholipid (PL) as shown in Fig. 5. Until middle age for rats (13 months old), there were no differences among control and GTC groups in terms of plasma lipids. At 19 months of age, the plasma lipids (TG, TC, PL) started to rise in all the dietary groups. Yet, the GTC group showed significant suppression of these parameters, particularly in plasma tryglyceride and total cholesterol concentrations. These data imply that as we age after maturity, it seems natural for the body to accumulate excess lipids. Yet, habitual intake of tea catechins seems to suppress an extreme accumulation of the lipids.

The importance of plasma cholesterol and lipoprotein concentrations in atherosclerosis has been noted by several researchers. Increased levels of plasma total cholesterol, in particular LDL cholesterol as well as the decrease of plasma HDL cholesterol are risk factors contributing to the development of coronary heart diseases (9). Our results suggest that catechins in green tea exert a hypocholesterolemic effect, and therefore have a protective effect against the atherosclerotic process. Massive oral doses of plant phenolic compounds (tannins) given to rats have been reported to cause growth depression and toxicity (10). In a separate experiment it was shown that slight growth depression occurred with 2% tea catechins added to the diet. One percent of tea catechins in the diet might be interpreted to be equivalent to 50–100 cups of green

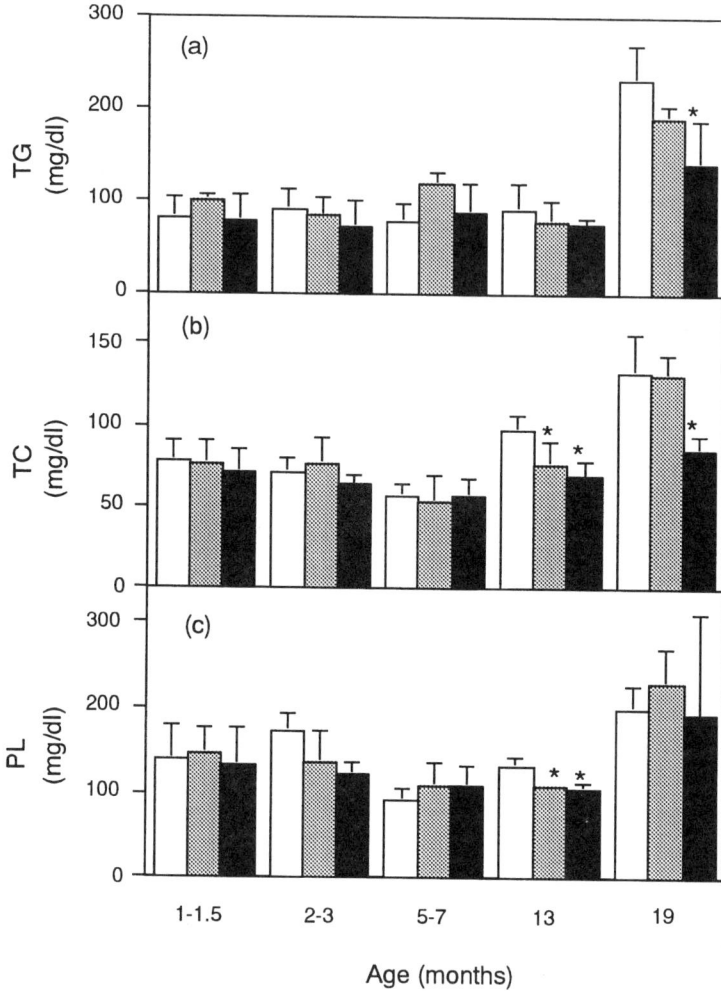

FIG. 5 Effects of dietary supplementation of GTC on the content of plasma lipids of rats. (a) TG, triglyceride; (b) TC, total cholesterol; (c) PL, phospholipid. Mean values + SD are given. Significantly different from the values of rats fed the basal diet. *p < 0.05. □: rats fed the basal diet. ▨: rats fed 0.5% GTC supplemented diet. ■: rats fed 1.0% GTC supplemented diet.

tea a day in the human diet. Therefore, any adverse effects on the human body by taking in an excessive amount of catechins are very unlikely.

IV. SUPPRESSION OF LDL OXIDATION BY TEA POLYPHENOLS

Oxidative modification of low-density lipoprotein (LDL) has been proposed to enhance its atherogenicity (11). It is quoted that antioxidants, such as vitamin E, provide resistance to this process (12) and that habitual intake of them will lower the incidence of coronary artery disease.

Dietary flavonoid intake has also been reported to be inversely associated with mortality from coronary artery disease (13). The low incidence of coronary artery disease in the French, who consume a high-fat diet (French paradox), has been attributed, in part, to regular consumption of red wine. In spite of the high smoking rate and susceptibility of oxidative modification of LDL in smokers, the mortality rates from coronary artery disease are much lower in China and in Japan than in the West (Far East paradox) where people drink a lot of tea. Tea polyphenols and red wine polyphenols are representative plant polyphenols that are consumed on a regular daily basis. Potent antioxidative properties of tea polyphenols have been described elsewhere. Ishikawa et al. (14) examined in vitro and in vivo the inhibitory effects of tea polyphenols on oxidative stress on LDL as follows.

A. In Vitro Study

Plasma was treated with tea polyphenols in order to adsorb them to LDL particles and the oxidizability of LDL isolated thereafter was measured. Blood collected from a normolipidemic healthy male volunteer was centrifuged to obtain serum. Tea catechins and theaflavins were mixed with serum in different concentrations (25 μM/L to 400 μM/L) and incubated for 3 hours at 37°C. Thereafter, LDLs were isolated from the serum by ultracentrifugation method and dialyzed for 12 hours at 4°C with degassed PBS (1L × 4 times) to obtain tea polyphenol-adsorbed LDL. Control LDL was treated without tea polyphenols. The oxidizability of LDL thus obtained was estimated by measuring three indexes (conjugated dienes, lipid peroxides and thiobarbituric acid reactive substances [TBARS]). By initiating the diene formation by Cu^{++}, the lag time before the oxidative propagation was measured as shown in Fig. 6. Galloyl catechins and theaflavins (EGCg, ECg, TF2 and TF3) increased lag time markedly and significantly before the onset of oxidative propagation in a dose dependent manner. Particularly, EGCg and TF3 prolonged lag time almost three times more than that of the control by 200 µM/L treatment, while vitamin E prolonged it only twice by 400 µM/L treatment (data not shown). Suppression of TBARS and lipid peroxides formation was also observed in the LDL samples with catechins (Fig. 7) and with theaflavins (Fig. 8). As shown in the figures, TBARS and lipid peroxide formation were sig-

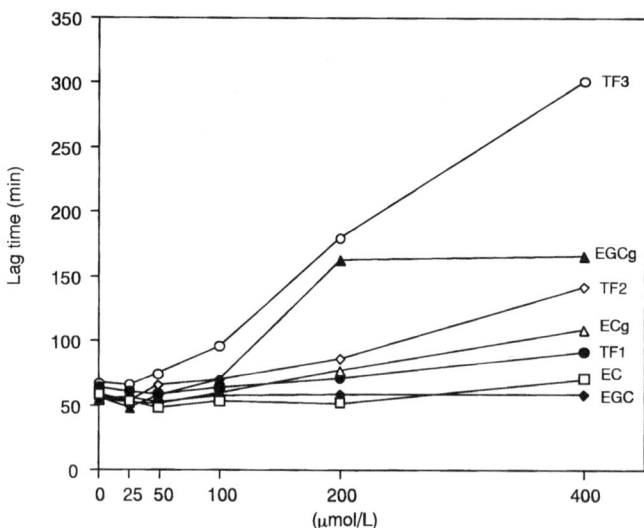

FIG. 6 Effect of in vitro addition of catechins (0-400 µM/L) to plasma on susceptibility of low-density lipoprotein to copper-induced oxidation.

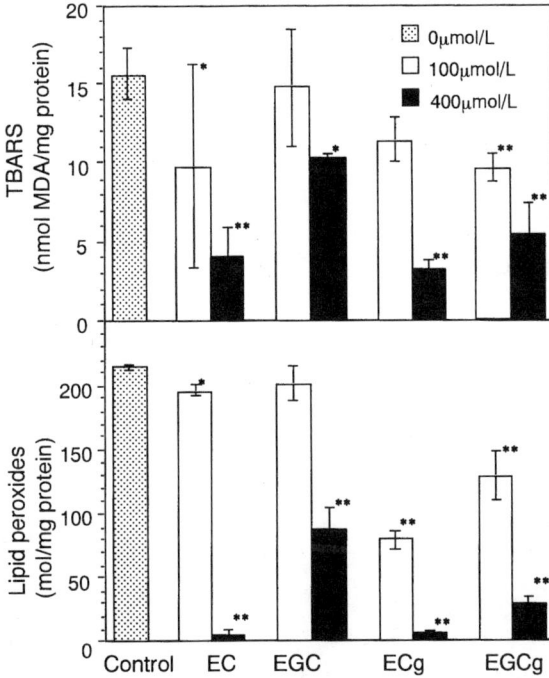

FIG. 7 Effect of in vitro addition of catechins to plasma on susceptibility of low-density lipoprotein to TBARS and macrophage-mediated oxidation. n = 4. One representative experiment of three is shown; the other two experiments yielded similar results. TBARS, thiobarbituric acid-reactive substance; MDA, malondialdehyde. TBARS and lipid peroxide differ significantly between groups, $p < 0.01$ (ANOVA).

Significantly different from control: *$p < 0.05$, **$p < 0.0001$.

nificantly reduced particularly in those LDL samples treated by 400μM/L tea polyphenols.

B. In Vivo Study

Normolipidemic healthy male volunteers (n = 22) aged 22 ± 1 years old, who abstained from tea for more than 4 weeks, were divided into two groups: tea and water. The tea group consumed five cups of black tea/day (11 g/750 mL/day) for four

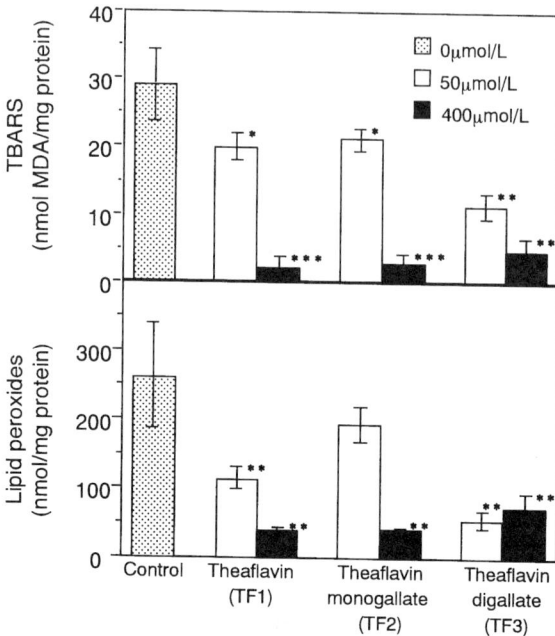

FIG. 8   Effect of in vitro addition of theaflavins to plasma on susceptibility of low-density lipoprotein to TBARS and macrophage-mediated oxidation. n = 4. One representative experiment of three is shown; the other two experiments yielded similar results. TBARS, thiobarbituric acid-reactive substance; MDA, malondialdehyde. TBARS and lipid peroxide differ significantly between groups, $p < 0.01$ (ANOVA).
   Significantly different from control: *$p < 0.05$, **$p < 0.01$, ***$p < 0.0001$.

weeks and the water group consumed the same amount of water. Blood samples were collected at the start and at the end of the study. After tea consumption for four weeks, significant prolongation of lag time before LDL oxidation was noted from 54 to 62 min, whereas no significant change was observed in the water group (Fig. 9). Other parameters showed no significant changes such as plasma total cholesterol, HDL cholesterol, triglyceride, apolipoprotein B, and plasma vitamin E between baseline and the end of the study in both groups.

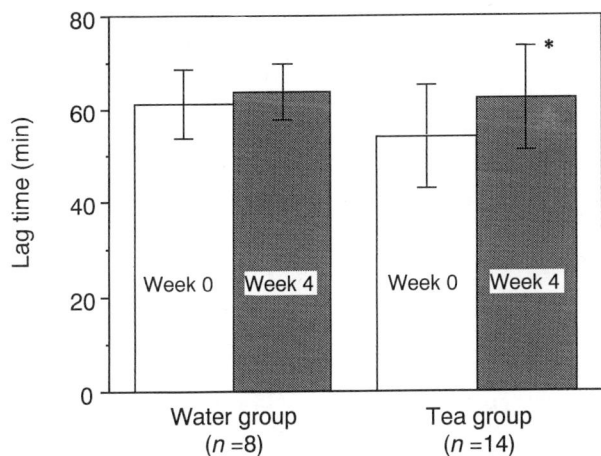

FIG. 9 Changes in oxidative susceptibility of low-denisty lipoprotein by black tea consumption in human volunteers. Significantly different from lag time at week 0, p < 0.01.

In a separate experiment, when 220 mg of EGCg was ingested in capsule form by a volunteer 1, 2, 3 h after ingestion, EGCg was present in the plasma at concentrations of 250, 230, and 180ηg/mL respectively. The concentration was highest 1 or 2 h after ingestion and had decreased slightly by 3 h after ingestion.

C. Discussion

In the in vitro experiment, oxidation of LDL that was isolated from plasma was significantly inhibited by preincubation with tea polyphenols in a dose-dependent manner. In the case of EGCg, ≥ 200 μM/L $\doteqdot$ 100 ηg/mL was necessary for a significant suppressive effect on LDL oxidizability.

Since only a part of EGCg seems to have been adsorbed to LDL and the rest was washed away, the effective amount of EGCg must be very trace in this experimental system. In the in vivo study, the mean lag time before LDL oxidation was significantly prolonged from 54 to 62 min after the subjects had consumed tea for four weeks, whereas no significant change was observed in the control group. The concentration of catechins in plasma was in the range of hundreds of ηg/mL a few hours after the ingestion, suggesting that a very similar situation will occur as it did in the in vitro experiment. Repeated exposure of LDL particles to tea polyphenols may enrich the LDL particles sufficiently to make them less susceptible to oxidative stress. Ascertaining the concentrations of tea polyphenols incorporated into LDL would contribute enormously to clarifying the mechanism by which tea affects LDL oxidizability. In conclusion, tea polyphenols may have favorable effects in ameliorating atherosclerosis by decreasing the susceptibility of LDL to oxidative modification.

V. SUPPRESSION OF THE ACCUMULATION OF BODY AND LIVER FAT

Male mice (13 weeks of age) were divided into three groups of eight animals. A diet of 5% palm oil was fed to the palm oil group (P_5). Palm oil is made mostly of saturated fatty acids. In addition to this diet, the catechin group was fed 0.1% GTC ($0.1GP_5$). Another group of mice was raised on the normal diet alone (N). Normal diet contained corn oil in the place of palm oil. Food and water were fed ad libitum. After three months, all mice were euthanized and their bodies and liver fat was measured by drying the carcasses (and organs) and extracting with ether.

Results showed that there were no significant differences in body weight gains or food intakes among the groups. As for the liver fat content, as shown in Fig. 10, the content elevated by palm oil (P_5) was suppressed by the addition of 0.1% GTC ($0.1GP_5$) to the same level as that of the normal diet (N). The same effect was shown in Fig. 11, where the body fat content elevated by palm oil was reduced to almost normal by the addition of 0.1% GTC. This amount (0.1% GTC) corresponds to 5–10 cups of tea per day. It is probable that the chances for obesity or fatty liver will be lessened by the habit of drinking

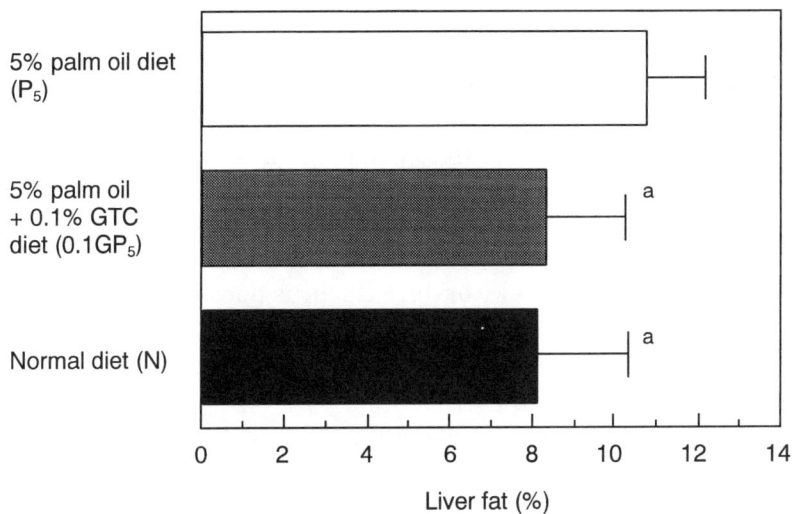

FIG. 10 Effect of catechin on liver fat of mice fed a high-fat diet for three months. a: $p < 0.05$ to P5.

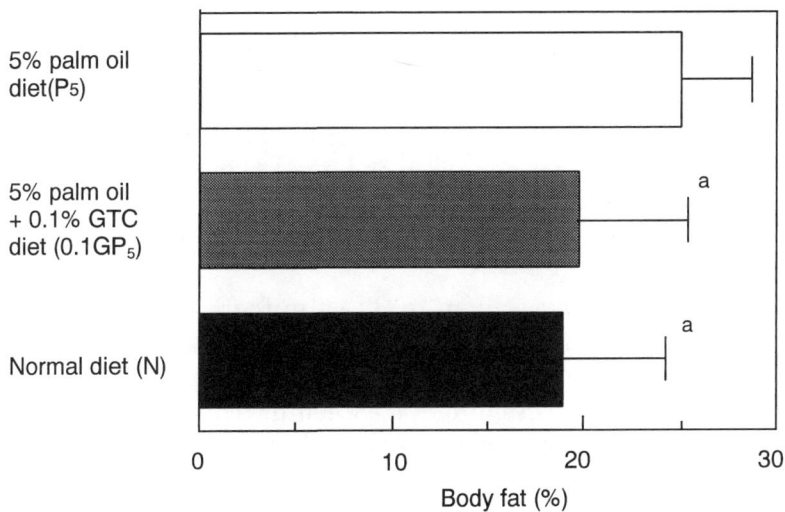

FIG. 11 Effect of catechin on body fat of mice fed a high-fat diet for three months. a: $p < 0.05$ to P5.

green tea. In a separate experiment, the reduction of liver and body fat by GTC was tried in the 15% palm oil diet but only a slight effect on the body fat was observed. In this case, the animal was a rat of five weeks of age and the test period was only one month. It seems that when the animal is in the process of growth, it is difficult to suppress the fat that is being built up inside the body. While we could expect the reduction of excessive bodily fat by tea catechins, it is also important to make sure that the intake of tea catechins does not also reduce any necessary fat in our bodies when we are eating a normal diet. We investigated this point in another experiment, where we found that although tea catechins were effective in suppressing the increase of body and liver fat in rats when fed for several months, there were no differences in body and liver fat among the test groups in the longer period feedings.

VI. HUMAN TRIALS

The influence of tea on plasma lipids was investigated by Iwata et al. in eighteen healthy young women, aged 18–20, who drank seven cups of oolong tea of average concentration daily for a period of six weeks (15). During the tea intake period, both triglyceride and phospholipid content decreased significantly, but two weeks after ceasing the tea intake, their respective concentrations returned to the initial levels. Although total cholesterol levels showed no change throughout the test period, HDL cholesterol levels increased significantly during the tea intake.

Tea catechin was given to 33 volunteers in the form of capsules (five capsules/day) for a period of three months. One capsule contained 100 mg of tea catechins which is equivalent to the average amount of catechins contained in 1–2 cups of tea of ordinary concentration. That is to say, the volunteers took 5–10 cups worth of catechins everyday for three months. As a result, their HDL cholesterol levels were elevated as shown in Fig. 12, though the total cholesterol levels remained unchanged. In another human trial, the levels of

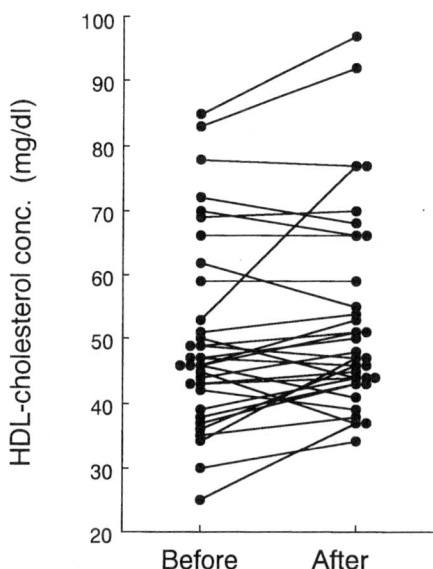

FIG. 12 HDL cholesterol levels in 33 volunteers taking 5 capsules (500 mg tea catechins) daily for three months.

LDL cholesterol showed a tendency to decrease when 1.5 grams of tea catechins were taken for three months by volunteers (data not shown).

REFERENCES

1. P Würsch. Influence of tannin-rich carob pod fiber on the cholesterol metabolism in the rat. J Nutr 109:685–692, 1979.
2. T Okuda, Y Kimura, T Yoshida, T Hatano, H Okuda, S Arichi. Studies on the activities of tannins and related compounds from medicinal plants and drugs. I. Inhibitory effects on lipid peroxidation in mitochondria and microsomes of liver. Chem Pharm Bull 31:1625–1631, 1983.
3. Y Fukuo. Serum lipoprotein metabolism in long-term users of high cholesterol diet (3 egg-yolks and green tea) [in Japanese]. Domyaku Koka, 10:981–988, 1982.
4. K Muramatsu, M Fukuyo, Y Hara. Effect of green tea catechins

on plasma cholesterol level in cholesterol-fed rats. J Nutr Sci Vitaminol 32:613–622, 1986.

5. M Fukuyo, Y Hara, K Muramatsu. Effect of Tea Leaf Catechin, (−)-epigallocatechin gallate, on plasma cholesterol level in rats [in Japanese]. Nihon Eiyo-Shokuryou Gakkaishi 39:495–500, 1986.

6. I Ikeda, Y Imasato, E Sasaki, M Nakayama, H Nagao, T Takeo, F Yayabe, M Sugano. Tea catechins decrease micellar solubility and intestinal absorption of cholesterol in rats. Biochimica et Biophysica Acta 1127:141–146, 1992.

7. N Matsumoto, K Okushio, Y Hara. Effect of black tea polyphenols on plasma lipids in cholesterol-fed rats. J Nutr Sci Vitaminol 44:337–342, 1998.

8. K Yoshino, I Tomita, M Sano, I Oguni, Y Hara, M Nakano. Effects of long-term dietary supplement of tea polyphenols on lipid peroxide levels in rats. Age 17:79–85, 1994.

9. T Gordon, WP Castelli, MC Hjortland, WB Kannel, TR Dawber. High density lipoprotein as a protective factor against coronary heart disease—the Framingham study. Am J Med 62:707–714, 1977.

10. JF Morton. Further associations of plant tannins and human cancer. Q J Cru Drug Res 12:1829–1841, 1971.

11. JL Witztum, D Steinberg. Role of oxidized low density lipoprotein in atherogenesis. J Clin Invest 88:1785–1792, 1991.

12. M Suzukawa, T Ishikawa, H Yoshida, H Nakamura. Effect of in vivo supplementation with low-dose vitamin E on susceptibility of low density lipoprotein and high-density lipoprotein to oxidative modification. J Am Coll Nutr 14:46–52, 1995.

13. MGL Hertog, EJM Feskens, PCH Hollman, MB Katan, D Kromhout. Dietary antioxidant flavonoids and risk of coronary heart disease: the Zutphen elderly study. Lancet 342:1007–1011, 1993.

14. T Ishikawa, M Suzukawa, T Ito, H Yoshida, M Ayaori, M Nishiwaki, A Yonemura, Y Hara, H Nakamura. Effect of tea flavonoid supplementation on the susceptibility of low-density lipoprotein to oxidative modification. Am J Nutr 66:261–266, 1997.

15. K Iwata, T Inayama, S Miwa, K Kawaguchi, G Koike. Effect of oolong tea on plasma lipids and lipoprotein lipase activity in young women [in Japanese]. Nihon Eiyou Shukuryou Gakkashi 44:251–259, 1991.

13

Hypoglycemic Action of Tea Polyphenols

I. INTRODUCTION

In our present society, obesity and diabetes are serious problems, both of which are bases for various complicated disorders. In both cases, well-programmed dietary control is crucial. In diabetes, ingested saccharides are not fully utilized as energy but stay in the bloodstream as glucose. A lack of insulin, the substance that keeps blood sugar levels within normal ranges, is a major cause of diabetes. Constantly higher concentrations of glucose in the blood renders the vein walls fragile and cause various disorders, such as renal failure, heart attacks, stroke, and high blood pressure. The eyes, kidneys, and nerves are prone to damage if diabetes is not carefully controlled. Control of diabetes requires correction of obesity, and a moderate intake of carbohydrates. Insulin injections are recommended for insulin dependent diabetes. Exercise may also aid in diabetes control. In obesity as well as in diabetes in particular, there are various dietary formulas recommended, the primary aim of these being to reduce the absorption of starch and sucrose. In any case, it is very desirable if daily drinking of tea or the intake of tea polyphenols can achieve this. Plant polyphenols are known to bind to proteins, and this property is utilized in the tanning of hide to make leather. The presence of plant polyphenols is also known to decrease the nutritional value of forage crops such as sorghum and various fodder tree leaves. Based on these properties, the inhibition of digestive enzymes such as α-amylase or sucrase by tea polyphenols was investigated.

II. IN VITRO ENZYME INHIBITION

Firstly, in vitro experiments were conducted (1,2). α-amylase and sucrase were chosen as α-glycosidase. As tea polyphenols, green tea catechins (EC, EGC, ECg, EGCg) and their stereo-isomers (C, GC, Cg, GCg), as well as black tea theaflavins (TF1, TF2A, TF2B, TF3), were tested for their enzyme inhibition. α-amylase of human saliva origin was used. The enzyme and starch were reacted in solution at 37°C for 10 min and α-amylase activity was determined by measuring the amount of separated maltose by colorimetric method. Crude sucrase was obtained by scraping the small intestinal mucosal brush border in rats. The crude sucrase and sucrose were reacted in solution at 37°C for 10 min and sucrase activity was determined by measuring the amount of glucose separated from sucrose by colorimetric method. Tea polyphenols at different concentrations were mixed in the above reaction solutions and the decreased amount of maltose (α-amylase) and glucose (sucrase) was compared with those of the controls. In the control, water was added in the place of tea polyphenol solution. The 50% inhibition dose (ID_{50}) was determined and is shown in Table 1 (α-amylase) and Table 2 (sucrase). As is apparent from Table 1, α-amylase was well inhibited by galloyl catechins (ECg, EGCg, Cg, GCg) and more strongly by theaflavins (TF1, TF2A, TF2B, TF3), but not by free catechins (EC, C, EGC,

TABLE 1   Inhibition of α-Amylase by Tea
Polyphenols and Gallic Acid

Sample	IC$_{50}$ (μM)
(−)-Epicatechin (EC)	>1000
(+)-Catechin (+C)	>1000
(−)-Epigallocatechin (EGC)	>1000
(−)-Gallocatechin (GC)	>1000
(−)-Epicatechin gallate (ECg)	130
(−)-Catechin gallate (Cg)	20
(−)-Epigallocatechin gallate (EGCg)	260
(−)-Gallocatechin gallate (GCg)	55
Theaflavin (TF1)	18
Theaflavin monogallate A (TF2A)	1.0
Theaflavin monogallate B (TF2B)	1.7
Theaflavin digallate (TF3)	0.6
Gallic acid	>1000

TABLE 2   Effect of Tea Polyphenols on Rat Small
Intestinal Sucrase

Sample	Concentration (mM)	Inhibition Activity (%)
None		0
Gallic acid	0.5	7
(+)-Catechin (+C)	0.5	14
(−)-Epicatechin (EC)	0.5	15
(−)-Epigallocatechin (EGC)	0.5	17
(−)-Epicatechin gallate (ECg)	0.5	62
(−)-Epicatechin gallate (ECg)	0.1	35
(−)-Epigallocatechin gallate (EGCg)	0.5	79
(−)-Epigallocatechin gallate (EGCg)	0.1	49
Theaflavin (TF1)	0.1	5
Theaflavin monogallate A (TF2A)	0.1	19
Theaflavin monogallate B (TF2B)	0.1	13
Theaflavin digallate (TF3)	0.1	42

GC). The 50% inhibitory concentrations of these compounds ranged from 0.6 ~ 260 μM.

In sucrase, galloyl catechins (ECg, EGCg) and theaflavin digallate (TF3) showed 35 ~ 50% inhibition at 0.1 mM which is much less than normal drinking concentrations. For both α-amylase and sucrase, free catechins (EC, EGC, C, GC) showed no noticeable inhibition. The mode of inhibition for both enzymes was noncompetitive. In the case of TF3 alone, it was a mixture of competitive and noncompetitive inhibition.

III. IN VIVO ANIMAL EXPERIMENTS

From the above results it was inferred that tea polyphenols might inhibit, in vivo, the digestion of starch and sucrose and suppress blood glucose levels. To verify this hypothesis, detailed hypoglycemic experiments were conducted with rats (3). Various amounts of green tea catechin (GTC) were administered to rats followed by a full but tolerable amount of saccharides 30 min afterward. At intervals over two hours after saccharide administration, plasma glucose and insulin concentrations, as well as intestinal enzyme activity, were measured.

Male wistar strain rats weighing 180 to 200 g (six weeks of age) were fed a commercial diet for one week. The rats were divided into four groups of 20 and starved overnight. GTC solutions of 80, 60, and 40 mg/ml were administered orally in 1 ml doses to each group of rats. Water was administered to the control group. After 30 min, 4 ml of 40% soluble starch solution was administered orally to all the rats. Immediately after administration and at 30 min, 1 hour, and 2 hour intervals, rats from all groups were killed and their blood was collected. The same procedure was followed for sucrose; with GTC solutions of 80, 10, and 5 mg/ml being administered to the test groups, followed by 4 ml of the 40% sucrose solution 30 min afterward. In order to see the effect of catechins on the digestion of glucose per se, one group of rats were administered glucose instead of starch or sucrose.

The results showed that when 80 or 60 mg of GTC were given 30 min before the administration of starch, the increase of glucose and insulin concentrations in the plasma was significantly suppressed as compared with those of the control group (Fig. 1). However, when 40 mg of GTC was given before starch administration, there was only slight suppression, demonstrating that suppression was dependent on the quantity of catechins administered to the rats. In the case of sucrose, 80 mg of GTC significantly suppressed the rise of glucose and insulin levels in the plasma which would otherwise have been elevated by sucrose (Fig. 2). Similar effects were observed with 10 mg of catechin administration, but no effect was observed with 5 mg of GTC. As expected, intestinal α-amylase activity of the catechin group (80, 60, and 40 mg) scarcely increased during the 2 hour period after administration of starch, but the enzyme activity of the control group increased markedly after the starch dosing (Fig. 3). In the same way, sucrase activity in the catechin groups (80, 10, and 5 mg) was significantly lower than that of the control group (Fig. 4). In the case of the glucose-administered group, the plasma glu-

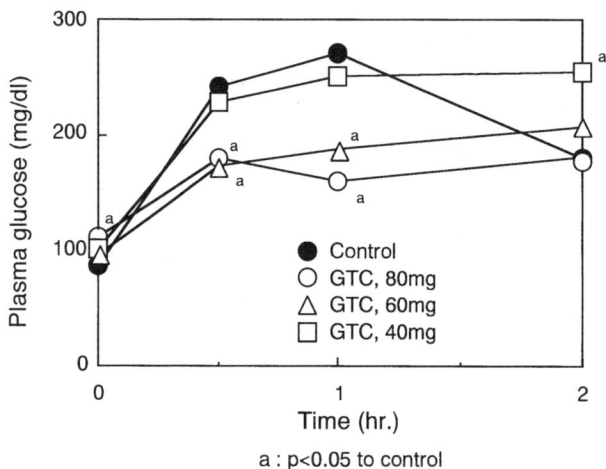

FIG. 1   Glucose concentration in blood plasma of rats administered starch.

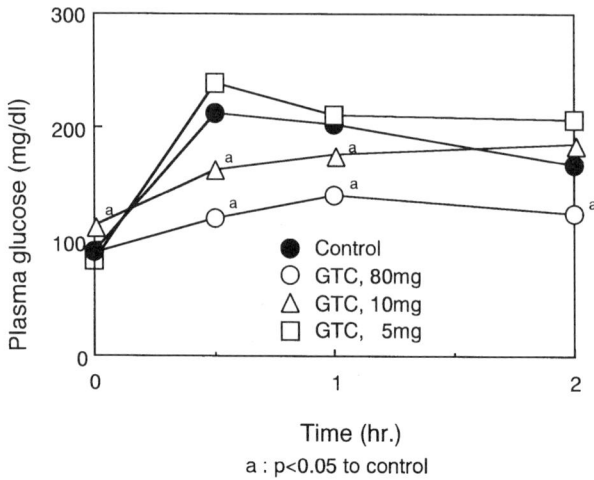

FIG. 2   Glucose concentration in blood plasma of rats administered sucrose.

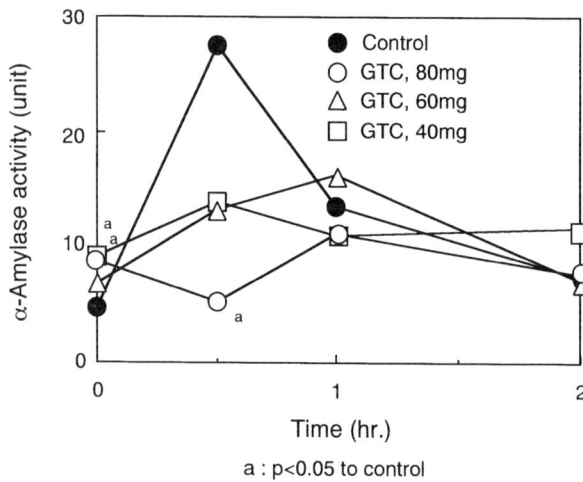

FIG. 3   α-Amylase activity in intestine of rats administered starch.

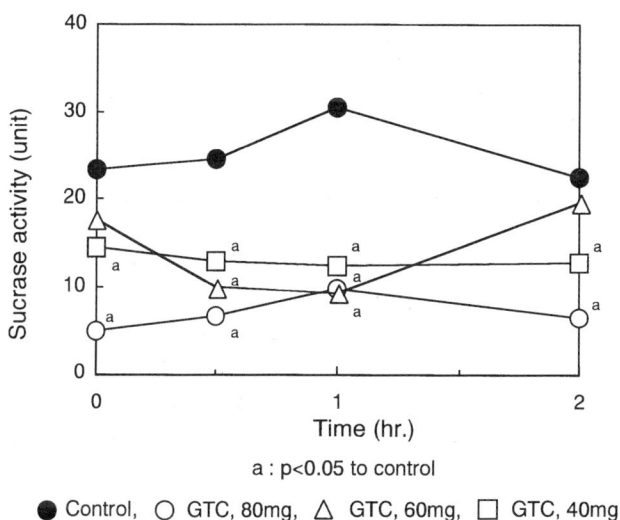

FIG. 4 Sucrase activity in intestine of rats administered sucrose.

cose level increased, regardless of whether catechin had been administered or not.

The results showed inhibition of α-amylase in the intestine, which was presumably responsible for the resultant suppression of plasma glucose and plasma insulin levels. There appears to be a certain threshold concentration for catechin to suppress plasma glucose levels. Simultaneous administration of starch with catechin had similar results (data not shown). Sucrase activity and plasma glucose levels were affected in the same way by prior or simultaneous administration of catechin with sucrose. The difference between the inhibition patterns of α-amylase and sucrase further indicates the interaction of these enzymes with catechin. As seen in Fig. 3, since α-amylase is secreted when starch enters the duodenum, there was hardly any difference between inhibition in the control and catechin-fed groups immediately after starch administration (0 min). At 30 min, when starch was present in the duodenum, enzyme activity peaked and was markedly inhibited by varying doses of catechin. On the other hand, sucrase is always present on the brush border membrane of the small intestine. Results in Fig. 4 show a definite inhibition of sucrase at 0 min, suggesting that the 30 min prior catechin dosing worked to suppress sucrase regardless of sucrose administration. Plasma insulin concentration increased proportionate to that of plasma glucose, and both were duly suppressed by catechins.

Throughout these experiments, it was postulated that inhibition of enzymes by tea polyphenols plays a key role in suppression of plasma glucose levels. Accelerated insulin secretion or the deterrence of glucose absorption from the bloodstream into the body, are other possible factors that can suppress increases in plasma glucose levels. However, it was confirmed in previous experiments that catechins have no influence on these factors (data not shown). In the same way, when glucose was given, catechin administration brought about no change in the pattern of plasma glucose level variations. It could be concluded from these experimental results that the inhibition of the above α-glycosidases by catechins was realized in the small intestine of rats and as a result, when a surfeit of starch or sucrose was administered, an increase in glucose levels was suppressed. In another series of experiments, it was confirmed that the amount of feces on a dry weight basis increased to nearly twice as much as that of the control in rats fed catechins over one month (4). This increase was found to gradually level off over a longer period of catechin feeding, indicating that there is a certain degree of supplemental secretion of α-amylase. It was also confirmed that as much as 1 or 2% catechin in the diet, fed over a period of three months, did not reduce body weight gains (Fig. 5) or food intakes (Fig. 6) as compared with those of control rats. These results indicate that the possible indigestibility of catechins would not cause any malnutrition. Detailed feeding experiments over a longer period are necessary to examine the influence of catechins on the absorption and excretion of carbohydrates in rodents as well as in humans.

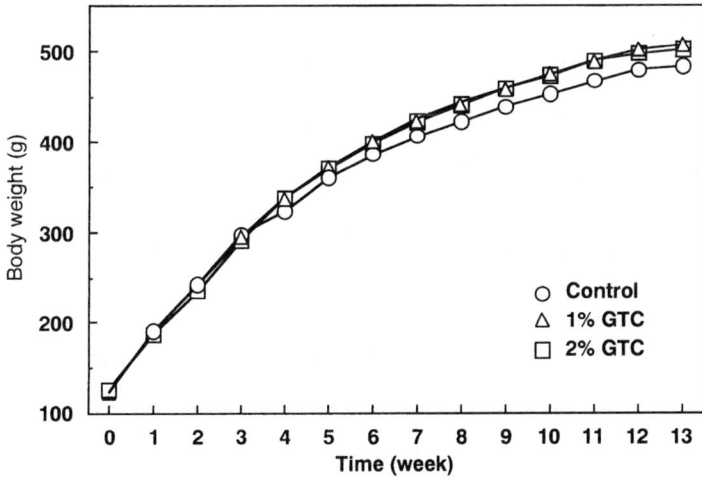

FIG. 5 The effect of GTC on body weight in rat fed diet containing GTC for three months.

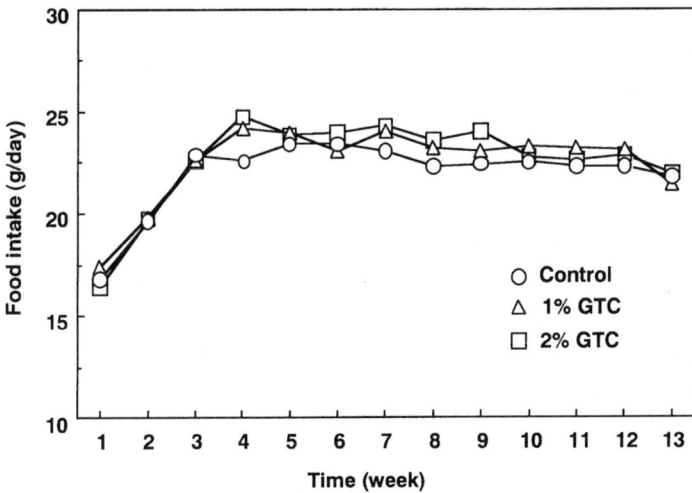

FIG. 6 The effect of GTC on food intake in rat fed diet containing GTC for three months.

REFERENCES

1. Y Hara, M Honda. The inhibition of α-amylase by tea polyphenols. Agric Biol Chem 54:1939–1945, 1990.
2. Y Hara, M Honda. Inhibition of rat small intestinal sucrase and α-glucosidase activities by tea polyphenols. Biosci Biotech Biochem 57:123–124, 1993.
3. N Matsumoto, F Ishigaki, A Ishigaki, H Iwashina, Y Hara. Reduction of blood glucose levels by tea catechin. Biosci Biotech Biochem, 57:525–527, 1993.
4. K Muramatsu, M Fukuyo, Y Hara. Effect of green tea catechins on plasma cholesterol level in cholesterol-fed rats. J Nutr Sci Vitaminol 32:613–622, 1986.

14

Hypotensive Action of Tea Polyphenols

I. INTRODUCTION

The following was quoted as one of the virtues of drinking tea at a seventeenth century tea house in London: "It helpth the headache, giddiness, and heavyness thereof (1)." In olden days there was no manometer to measure blood pressure, yet the above quotation implies that tea drinking might have alleviated headaches, giddiness, and heaviness caused by hypertensive circulation in the brain.

II. INHIBITION OF HYPERTENSIVE ENZYME

Most hypertension in humans occurs as essential hypertension, and compounds of the renin-angiotensin system are said to play a large role. As shown in Fig. 1, angiotensinogen, a kind of glycoprotein, is discharged into the bloodstream from the liver. Angiotensinogen is converted to angiotensin I by renin, an enzyme produced in the kidneys. Angiotensin I, a deca-

ASP-ARG-VAL-TYR-ILE-HIS-PRO-PHE-HIS-LEU-LEU-VAL-TYR-SER ....   (Angiotensinogen)

↓ Renin (Kidney)

ASP-ARG-VAL-TYR-ILE-HIS-PRO-PHE-HIS-LEU   (Angiotensin I)

↓ Converting enzyme (Lung)

ASP-ARG-VAL-TYR-ILE-HIS-PRO-PHE   (Angiotensin II)

↓ "Angiotensinases"

Inactive products

+

ARG-VAL-TYR-ILE-HIS-PRO-PHE   (Angiotensin III)

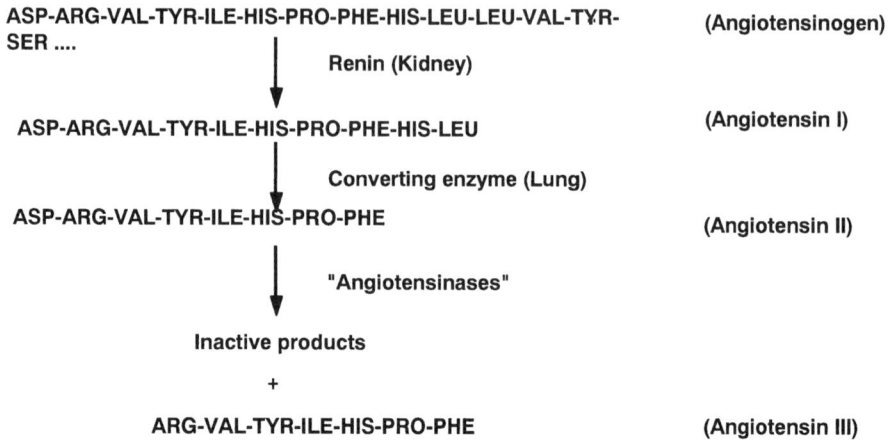

FIG. 1   The renin-angiotensin system. Angiotensin I-converting enzyme cleaves the carboxyl terminal end of the inactive decapeptide angiotensin I to form the potent vasopressor octapeptide angiotensin II.

peptide that is inactive, is then converted to angiotensin II by the enzyme ACE (angiotensin I converting enzyme). The main site of this reaction is the lungs. The resultant angiotensin II, an octapeptide, circulates throughout the whole vascular system and exerts severe vasoconstriction on the microcirculation system. Consequently, an effective therapy for hypertension could be achieved by suppressing the action of ACE. Based on this hypothesis, various kinds of ACE inhibitors were synthesized and captopril is now used clinically worldwide to treat hypertensive patients. In vitro experiments may be done using Hip-His-Leu solution in place of angiotensin I and the amount of His-Leu cleaved by the addition of ACE is compared with the amount cleaved in a solution to which the inhibitor has been mixed . Suzuki et al. screened the ACE inhibiting ability of the extracts of 117 kinds of foods consumed daily as well as those of Chinese medicinal herbs (2). Infused tea showed rather potent inhibition as did extracts of buckwheat, clams, some fruits, and soybeans, among others. We

TABLE 1   Inhibitory Effects of Tea Polyphenols Against
Angiotensin I Converting Enzyme (ACE)

Tea Polyphenols	Inhibition (IC_{50})
(−)-Epicatechin gallate (ECg)	1400 µM
(−)-Epigallocatechin gallate (EGCg)	90
Theaflavin (TF1)	400
Theaflavin monogallate A (TF2A)	115
Theaflavin monogallate B (TF2B)	110
Theaflavin digallate (TF3)	35
(Captopril	0.078)

have investigated the component in tea that exerts ACE inhibition. The results, as given in Table 1, show that tea polyphenols, such as EGCg and TF3 were fairly potent in inhibiting ACE. There are three active sites in ACE: the Zn^{++} site, hydrogen bonding site, and the positively charged site as shown in Fig. 2. EGCg will interact with these sites, thus inhibiting the approach of angiotensin I to these sites.

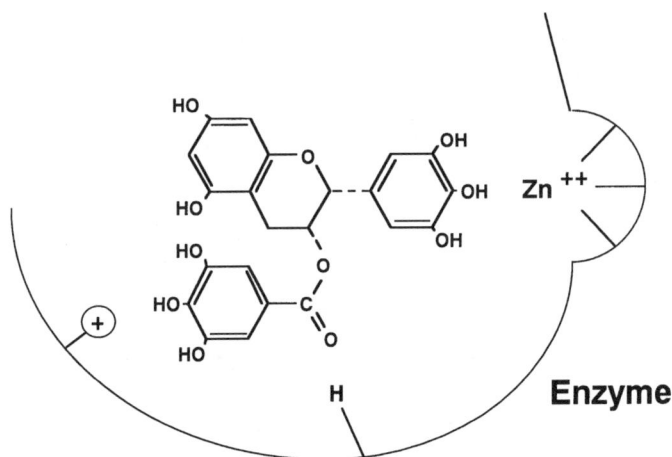

FIG. 2   Possible interaction of EGCg with the active site of ACE.

III. ANIMAL EXPERIMENTS

In the next step, we investigated the hypotensive effect of tea polyphenols on animals. Spontaneously hypertensive rats (SHR) are specially genetically bred rats that develop hypertension as they grow. This strain is used as a model for human hypertension. The SHRs were divided into two groups. The first group received a normal diet, while the second group was given a diet containing 0.5% green tea catechin (GTC) powder from one week after weaning. Although the blood pressure in the normal diet group already exceeded 200 mmHg at 10 weeks of age, significant suppression was noted in the 0.5 % GTC group (Fig. 3). When the diet of both groups was switched at 16 weeks of age, the blood pressures, in time, also changed accordingly, as shown in the Fig. 3. These results and other trials revealed that when the rats were fed catechins at an age later than weaning, it was difficult to suppress hypertension

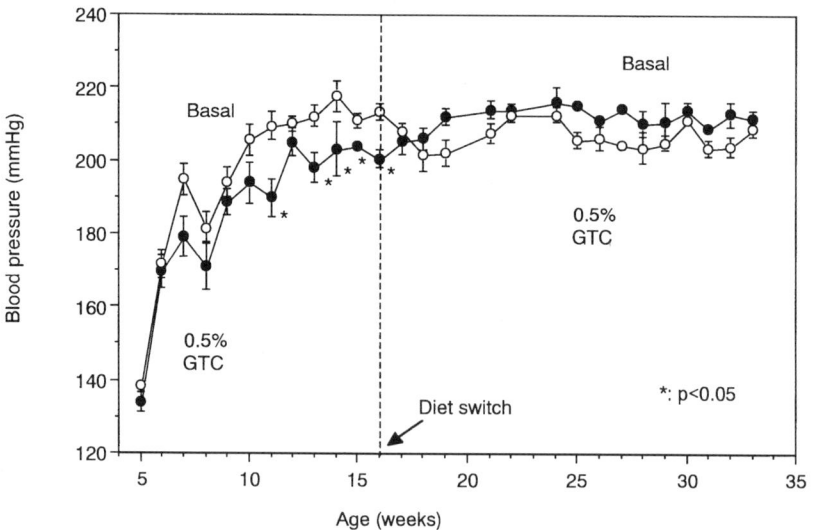

FIG. 3   Effect of green tea catechins (GTC) on blood pressure of SHR (spontaneously hypertensive rats).

significantly against the control group, yet it was noted that feeding of catechins at a later age did tend to suppress hypertension, although not significantly. In the course of these experiments, we realized that to obtain duplicable results on blood pressure using the plethysmometry method (measuring the pressure of the bloodstream of the tail) requires dexterity on the part of the researcher and affinity with the animals in the experiment. In order to confirm hypotensive potency of tea polyphenols on a more solid basis, we observed the death rate of stroke-prone SHR (SHRSP) and used this as an index. In order to accelerate the outbreak of brain stroke, 1% salt was added to the drinking water. During the feeding period of 16 weeks before the mice began to die from brain stroke, there were no differences in body weight gain or food intake between the normal diet group and the catechin diet group. As shown in Fig. 4, the catechin-fed group tended to have lower blood pressure during this period as compared with the normal diet group. Fig. 5 shows the death curves of brain strokes. As shown in the figure, addition of 0.5% GTC delayed the out-

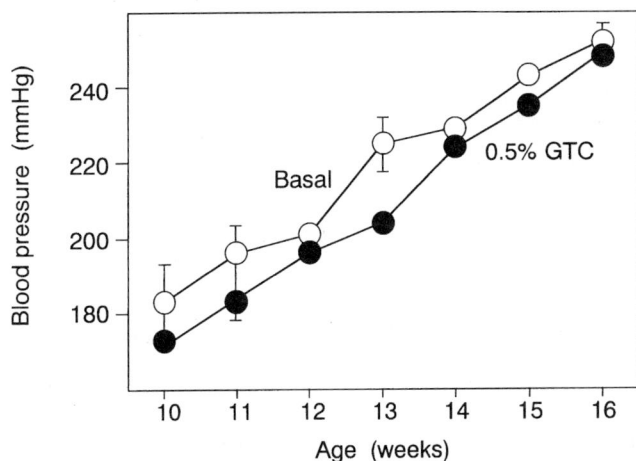

FIG. 4   Effect of GTC on blood pressure of SHRSP (stroke-prone SHR).

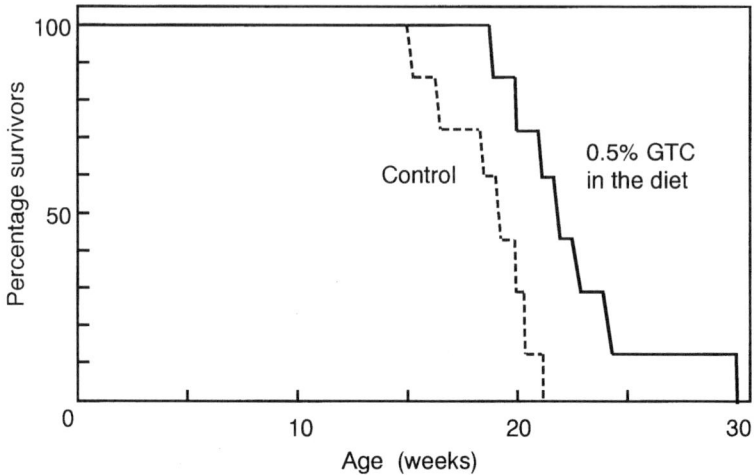

FIG. 5   Effect of GTC on the lifespan of SHRSP.

break of stroke and extended the lifespan of the rats more than 15% as compared with the control group. These results implied that tea might be effective in preventing hypertension in humans.

IV.   HUMAN TRIALS

Human trials were conducted to confirm the effect of catechins on 21 volunteers. They received a total of 500 mg of tea catechins (in capsule form) a day, administered twice daily after breakfast and lunch for 12 weeks. The results in Fig. 6 show that administration of catechins lowered blood pressure significantly for both the systolic (from 134 ± 14.8 mmHg to124.5 ± 17.6 mmHg) and the diastolic (from 84.5 ± 9.8 mmHg to 76.6 ± 11.0 mmHg) readings; moreover, a nutritional survey revealed improvement in general condition. In particular, bowel movement regularity improved considerably in the subjects.

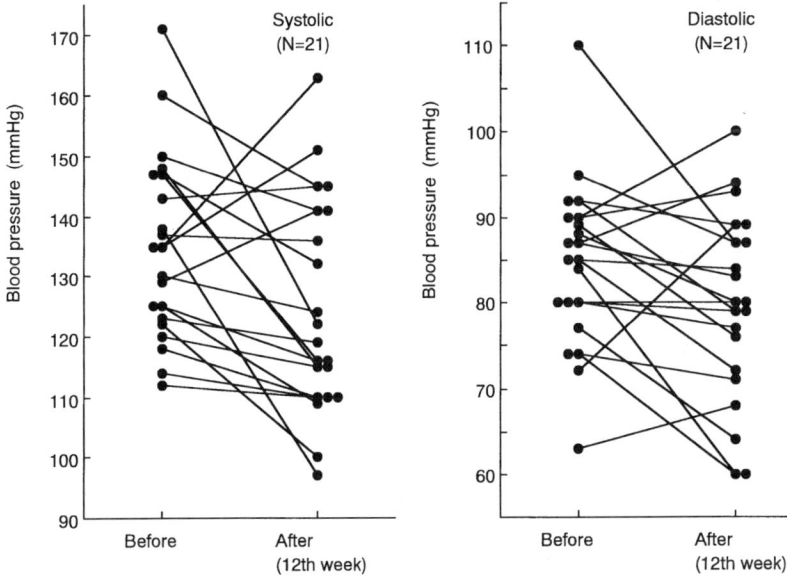

FIG. 6   Effect of dietary tea catechins (500 mg/day) on blood pressure in 21 volunteers.

V.   EPIDEMIOLOGICAL DATA

Sato et al. studied the epidemiological consequences of tea drinking on brain stroke among 9,510 human subjects (3). These subjects were all women over age 40, all nonsmokers and nondrinkers, and were selected from an initial group of 31,769 subjects surveyed. To avoid any possible confounding factors, smokers and drinkers were eliminated from the study, leaving no male subjects in the final study group. Questionnaires were completed by the subjects regarding their history of brain stroke. As shown in Fig. 7, those who were in the habit of drinking more than five cups of tea a day had a lesser chance of brain stroke, regardless of other factors such as daily salt intake, age, and environment (urban or rural). These data

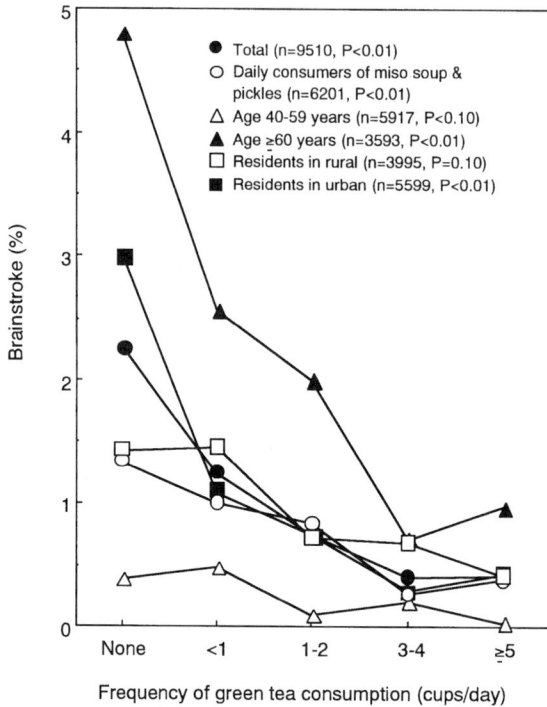

FIG. 7   Effect of green tea composition on the reduction of brain stroke history. Nonsmoking and nondrinking women aged 40 and over were studied.

imply that drinking a considerable amount of tea daily will lessen our chances of brain stroke.

VI.   GABARON TEA

An entirely new process of tea manufacturing was proposed by Tsushida (4). The resultant new tea was found to have a greater hypotensive effect than conventionally produced teas. In this new process freshly plucked tea leaves are incubated in inert gas (e.g., nitrogen or carbon dioxide) for more than a few hours. Thereafter, the conventional tea manufacturing process for green tea, black tea, or oolong tea is followed. Dur-

ing this anaerobic treatment, leaf cells that remain alive undergo specific metabolism on their own and develop a fair
amount of γ-amino butyric acid (GABA). GABA is formed from
glutamic acid by enzymatic decarboxylation. Usually tea, both
green or black, contains less than 20 mg% of GABA. Gabaron
tea accumulates more than 150 mg%—or sometimes 200
mg%—of GABA in the processed dry leaves. At the same time
gabaron tea develops a particular flavor, slightly similar to
that of pickles, which distinguishes this tea from the conventional ones. After all, anaerobic treatment is biochemically
much like that of pickle production. This particular flavor is
weakened by additional light roasting of the gabaron tea after
the completion of the usual tea manufacturing process. Omori
et al. gave gabaron green tea extract (5 g/100 ml hot water,
1 min) to six-week-old spontaneously hypertensive rats
(SHRs) as drinking water for 18 weeks (5). Ordinary green

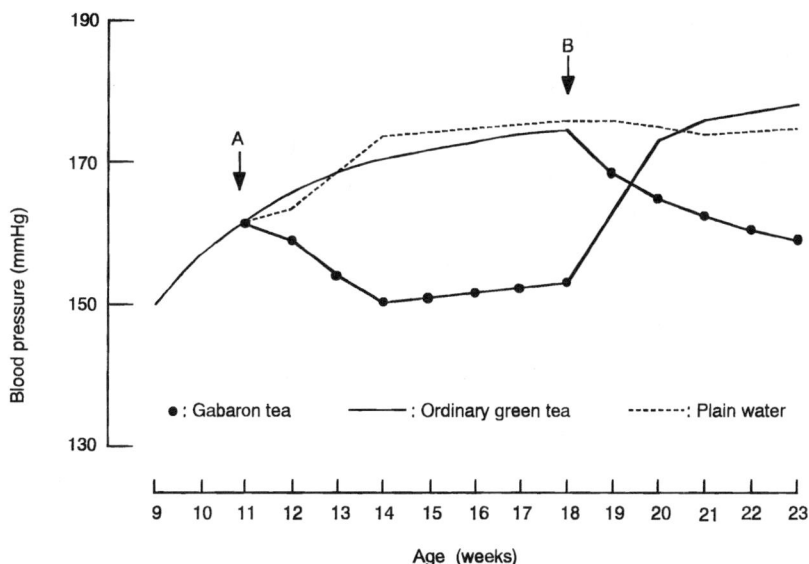

FIG. 8 Effect of gabaron tea on blood pressure in rats (SHR). (A) Before
administration; (B) after administration.

tea extract and plain water were fed as controls (each group consisted of eight rats). As shown in Fig. 8, after commencing feeding of gabaron tea extract at the 11th week, the systolic blood pressure of the test group tended to be lower than the other groups. When the drinking water was changed between the gabaron group and the ordinary tea group, the blood pressure curve changed accordingly.

REFERENCES

1. WH Ukers. All About Tea. New York: The Tea and Coffee Trade Journal Company, 1935.
2. T Suzuki, N Ishikawa, H Meguro. Angiotensin I-converting enzyme inhibiting activity in foods (studies on vasodepressive components in foods. Part I) [in Japanese]. Nippon Nogeikagaku Kaishi 57:1143–1146, 1983.
3. Y Sato, H Nakatsuka, T Watanabe, S Hisamichi, H Shimizu, S Fujisaku, Y Ichinowatari, Y Ida, S Suda, K Kato, M Ikeda. Possible contribution of green tea drinking habits to the prevention of stroke. Tohoku J Exp Med 157:337–343, 1989.
4. T Tsushida, T Murai. Conversion of glutamic acid to γ-aminobutyric acid in tea leaves under anaerobic conditions. Agric Biol Chem 51:2865–2871, 1987.
5. M Omori, T Yano, J Okamato, T Tsushida, T Murai, M Higuchi. Effect of anaerobically treated tea (gabaron tea) on blood pressure of spontaneously hypertensive rats [in Japanese]. Nippon Nogeikagaku Kaishi 61: 1449–1451, 1987.

15

Effects on Intestinal Flora

I. INTRODUCTION

A human intestine harbors 100 trillion viable bacteria of 100 different species which form the intestinal flora. The condition of the intestinal flora influences many factors pertaining to the host's health and vise versa. These factors include, as shown in Fig. 1, infection, immune response, cancer, aging, physiological function, effect of medicine, and nutrition. While the intestinal flora is made up of beneficial, detrimental, or nondescript bacteria, a satisfactory balance thereof may be achieved by a nutritionally well-balanced diet. Moreover, active intake of a diet which promotes useful bacteria and suppresses harmful bacteria, such as oligosaccharide, dietary fiber, or fermented milk is recommended. Since tea polyphenols (green tea catechins and black tea polyphenols) show specific antibacterial effects against floral bacteria and the majority of tea polyphenols are considered to remain in the intestine

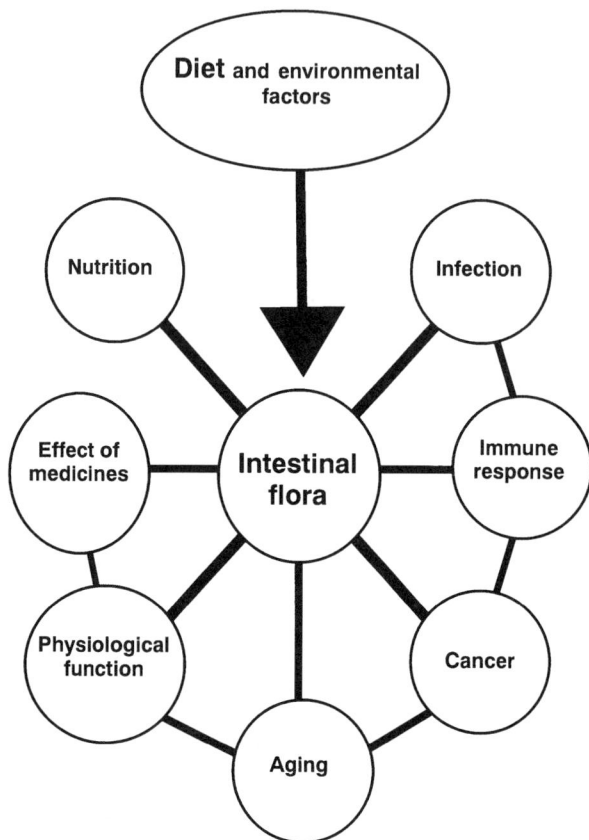

FIG. 1 Influence of intestinal flora on the host. (Original: Tomotari Mitsuoka)

before being excreted in the feces, their influence on human intestinal flora is of great interest.

II. EFFECTS OF TEA CATECHINS ON INTESTINAL FLORA AND THE REDUCTION OF FECAL ODOR

While tea polyphenols were proven *in vitro* to have strong antibacterial action against harmful foodborne pathogenic bacteria, this same action was not observed against lactic acid bacteria such as lactobacillus or bifidobacterium, which are regarded as playing a beneficial role in the maintenance of the healthy intestinal flora (Table 1). In another series of experiments, we have confirmed that more than 50% of orally ingested catechins are excreted via feces, indicating that the majority of tea catechins ingested pass through the intestinal flora (1). Hence, the influence of tea polyphenols on the condition of the intestinal flora of the large intestine is of great interest. In the following experiments, we have confirmed remarkable improvement in bowel conditions in animals as well as in humans by the administration of tea catechins equivalent to only 5–6 cups/day of tea.

A. Marked Improvement of Intestinal Conditions and Reduction of Fecal Odors of Elderly People

In this study, the effects of tea catechins on fecal flora and fecal metabolic products were investigated in elderly inpatients who were being fed by nasal tube in health care centers (2). Fecal odor is one of the biggest problems in nursing homes. The odor of the residents' feces is unpleasant and makes the caretaker's job difficult at times. Lessening the odor would improve the environment of nursing homes where many aged people live together.

The feces of healthy adults have bacterial concentrations of about 300–500 billion, including more than 100 species per gram. They are mainly composed of anaerobes such as *Bacteroidaceae*, eubacteria, *Peptococcaceae* and bifidobacteria, as well as intestinal aerobic bacteria. Maintaining good condition of the intestinal flora is considered to be important not only in maintaining bowel regularity, but also for keeping the body in good condition generally through metabolic activity. However, concomitantly with the onset of old age, characteristic changes in fecal flora appear; that is, decreasing numbers of bifidobacteria and increasing numbers of putrefying bac-

TABLE 1 Minimum Inhibitory Concentrations of Tea Catechins Against Foodborne Pathogenic and Enteric Bacteria

Bacteria	MIC (ppm)				
	GTC	EC	ECg	EGC	EGCg
Staphylococcus aureus IAM 1011	450	> 800	800	150	250
Vibrio fluvialis JCM 3752	200	800	300	300	200
V. parahaemolyticus IFO 12711	200	800	500	300	200
V. metschnikovii IAM 1039	500	>1000	>1000	500	1000
Clostridium perfringens JCM 3816	400	>1000	400	1000	300
C. botulinum A, B mix.	< 10	>1000	200	300	< 100
Bacillus cereus JCM 2152	600	>1000	600	>1000	600
Plesiomonas shigelloides IID No. 3	100	700	100	200	100
Aeromonas sobria JCM 2139	400	>1000	700	400	300
Lactobacillus brevis subsp. gravesensis JCM 1102	>1000	>1000	>1000	>1000	>1000
L. brevis subsp. *brevis* JCM 1059	>1000	>1000	>1000	>1000	>1000
L. brevis subsp. *otakiensis* JCM 1183	>1000	>1000	>1000	>1000	>1000
Bifidobacterium bifidum JCM 1255	>1000	>1000	>1000	>1000	>1000
B. adolescentis JCM 1275	>1000	>1000	>1000	>1000	>1000
B. longum JCM 1217	>1000	>1000	>1000	>1000	>1000

GTC: Green Tea Catechin, EC: (−)-epicatechin, ECg: (−)-epicatechin gallate, EGC: (−)-epigallocatechin, EGCg: (−)-epigallo-catechin gallate.

teria such as *Enterobacteriaceae*, enterococci, and clostridia appear.

The subjects of the study were 10 females and 5 males, from 51 to 93 years of age (average 70.3). None of the subjects had conditions related to the gastrointestinal tracts or endocrine organs. All subjects received the same daily diet, 1000 kcal of gastroenteral liquid alimentation, supplemented with 300 mg of tea catechins (in the form of Polyphenon 60™, 484 mg), which was divided into three doses and dissolved in the liquid alimentation immediately before administration three times a day. The daily tea catechin administration was equivalent to that contained in about 5–6 cups of green tea. Daily tea catechin administration was continued for a period of three weeks. Fecal specimens were collected at the end of the first, second, and third week after administration as well as just before and one week after. Favorable results were obtained with regards to not only fecal flora and fecal metabolic products, but also with regard to odor and volume increase of feces.

In comparison of the values before administration with those during tea catechin administration, levels of lactobacilli and bifidobacteria increased significantly with the administration of catechins, whereas the levels of *Enterobacteriaceae* decreased. The detection rate of lecithinase-positive and -negative clostridia showed a tendency to decrease during administration. The levels of lecithinase-negative clostridia decreased significantly. The levels of total bacteria, *Bacteroidaceae*, and eubacteria, decreased significantly (Fig. 2). Meanwhile, the levels of coagulase-negative staphylococci increased. Fecal concentrations of ammonia during administration decreased significantly. Fecal concentrations of sulfide increased initially, but then also decreased significantly (Fig. 3). The amount of total fecal organic acids increased significantly whereas pH values decreased (Fig. 4). Fecal phenol, cresol, ethylphenol, indole, and skatol decreased significantly (Fig. 5). Fecal ammonia, sulfide, and odorous metabolites are responsible for the offensive odor of feces and the decreases in their

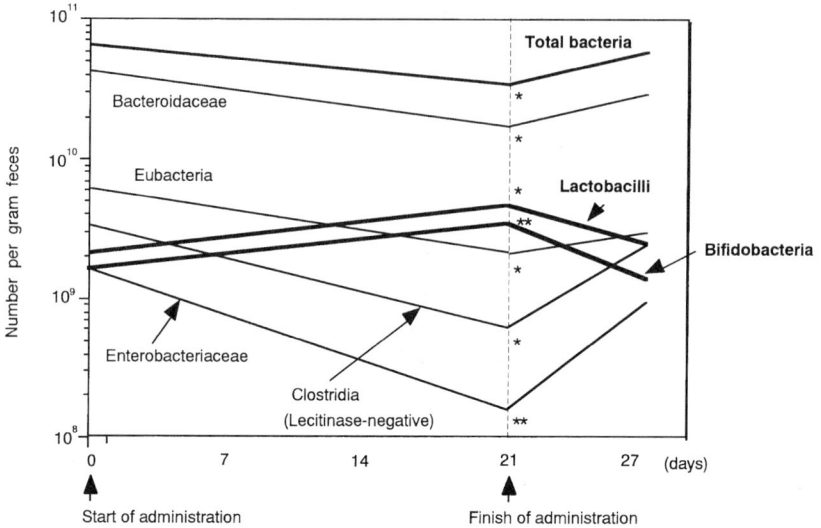

FIG. 2 Effect of P-60 administration on fecal flora of 15 human volunteers (300 µg tea catechins/day). Graph is expressed as mean ± SD. Significant differences (* = $p < 0.05$, **$p < 0.01$, *** = $p < 0.001$) from value of day 0 (before the administration).

levels in the feces of subjects receiving tea catechin supplements corresponded to observations by nursing staff who reported a reduction of fecal odor in 11 cases out of 15 subjects. The reduction in fecal odor is a positive factor when considering the role of caregivers and the comfort of their patients. It was also noted that there was a tendency for the volume of feces to increase during tea catechin administration. This increase might have been caused by the property of tea catechins to inhibit the action of α-amylase (3).

In a recent follow-up study, we administered catechins, according to the same protocol as above, to 35 elderly residents in a long-term care facility who were all on the same gruel diet. Catechins were given in the form of tablets. The fecal parameters showed almost identical tendencies as the previous experiment, thus endorsing the beneficial effects of tea catechins on bowel conditions (4).

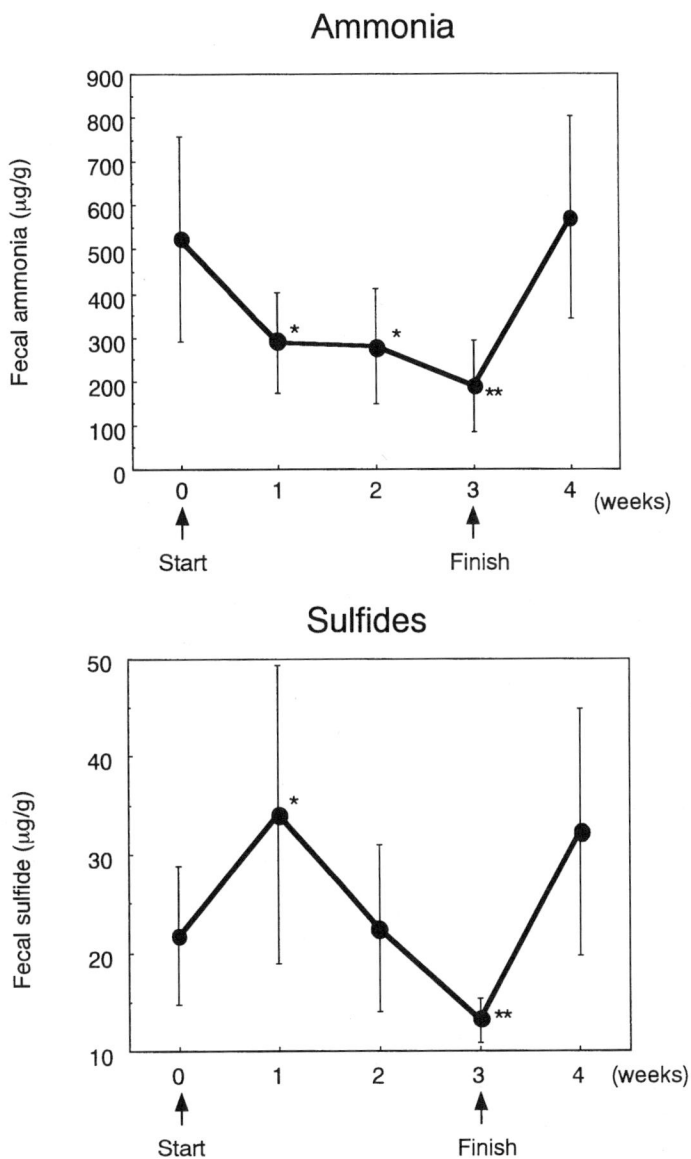

FIG. 3 Effect of P-60 on fecal ammonia and sulfide in humans.

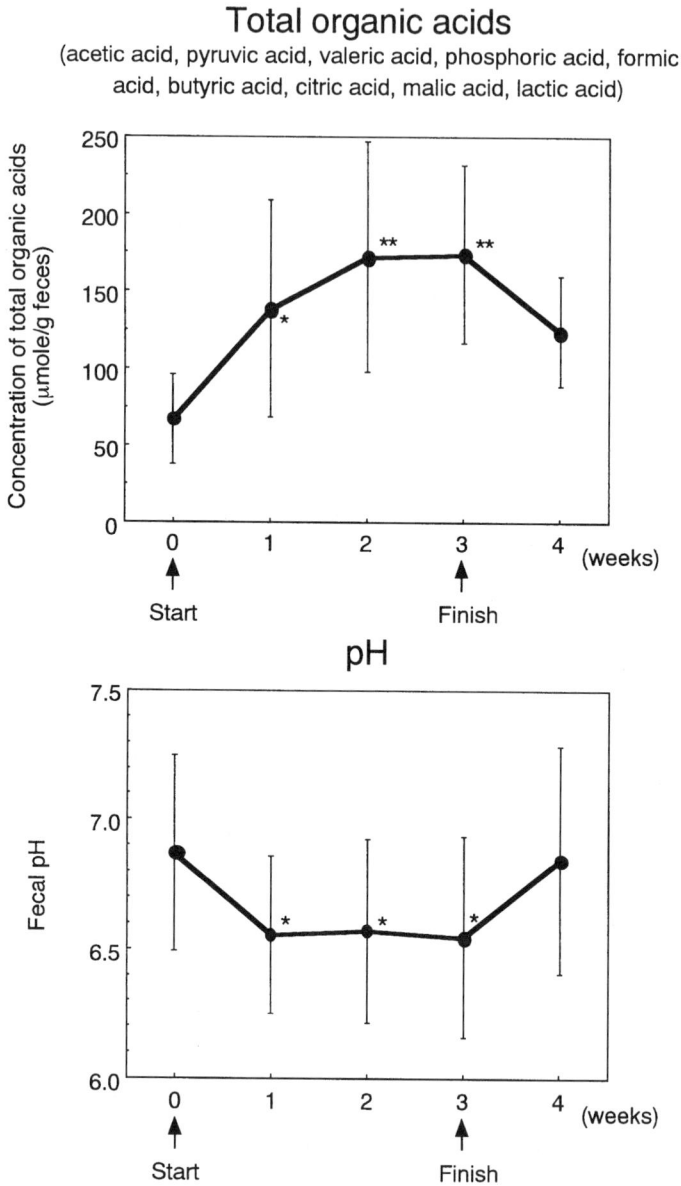

FIG. 4   Effect of P-60 on fecal organic acids and pH in humans.

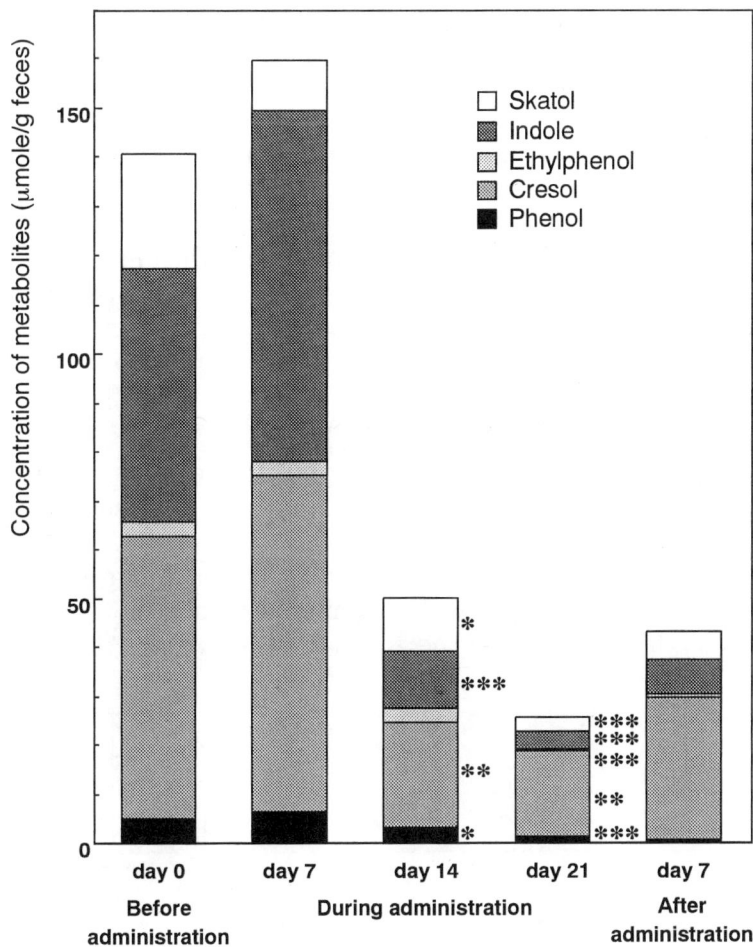

FIG. 5 Effect of tea catechin administration on fecal metabolites of 15 human volunteers. Significant differences (*p = 0.05, **p < 0.01, ***p < 0.001) from the value of day 0 (before administration).

Previously, we carried out similar tests on six volunteers, not under hospitalization, who received 500 mg of tea catechins everyday for 30 days. We monitored fecal pH, ammonia, and fecal flora and noted no statistically significant changes after catechin dosing, most probably because of the big daily differences in diet of the subjects (data not shown).

The results indicate that tea polyphenols may work to reverse conditions in fecal flora associated with the onset of old age by maintaining a healthy balance between the flora's acid producing bacteria and putrefactive bacteria. This is relevant not only for hospital patients but for the general population.

III. BOWEL MOVEMENTS OF HUMANS

In a group of 37 volunteers, similar positive effects of polyphenols were observed (5). Five catechin capsules (in total 500 mg of catechins) were ingested daily for a period of 12 weeks. It was discovered that while just about 50% of the group reported to have regular bowel movements before the experiment (i.e., the other half of the group were irregular), that fig-

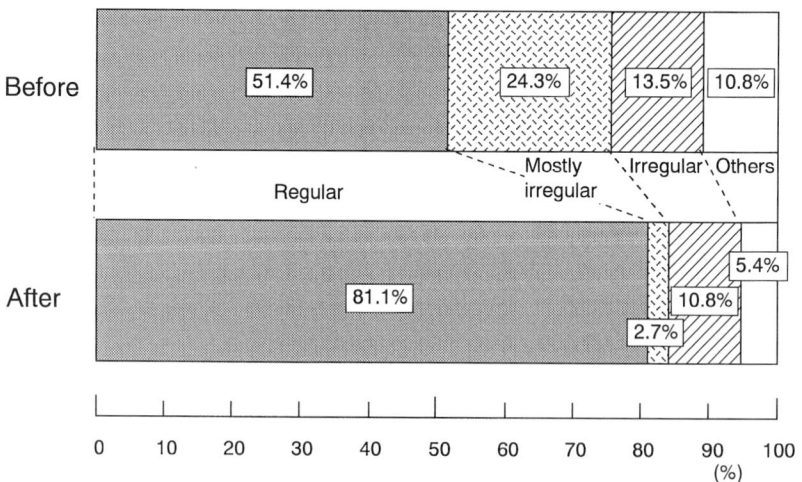

FIG. 6   Effect of tea catechin ingestion (500 mg/day/3 mo.) on bowel movement habitude in humans (N = 37).

ure rose to just over 80% on completion of the polyphenol supplemented diet (Fig. 6). All of those interviewed reported the favorable improvement of their bowel conditions.

IV. EFFECT OF TEA CATECHINS ON INTESTINAL FLORA OF CHICKENS

Broiler chickens were divided into two groups (each 10,000) and one group was fed a diet containing 0.07% tea catechins, while the other group was fed a regular diet for a period of 61 days from the first day of hatching (6). On the 56th day, eight chicks per group were killed and cecal samples were collected for analysis.

On analysis of the ceca of the chickens from each group, significant differences were observed in the catechin-fed group as compared to the control group. In the flora, *Lactobacilli* increased significantly ($10^{8.6} \rightarrow 10^{9.4}$/gram) whereas *Enterobacteriaceae* decreased significantly ($10^{9.4} \rightarrow 10^{8.8}$/gram). Another notable change was the significant decrease of the detection rate for proteus, which produces malodorous compounds from protein, although the total number of bacteria did not change

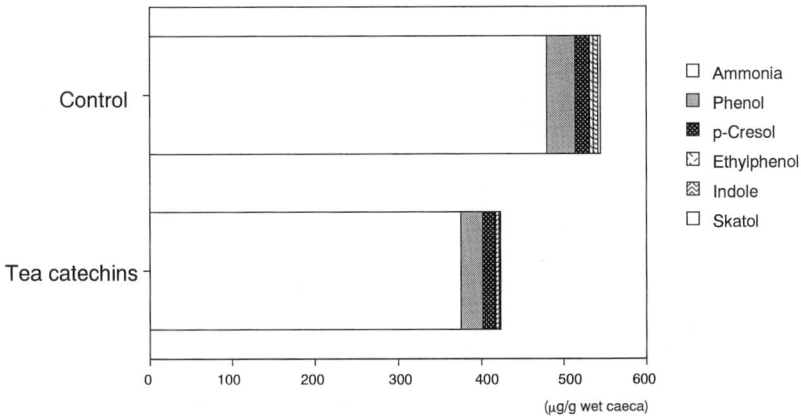

FIG. 7   Effect of tea catechin administration (0.07% of diet) on caecal putrefactive products of chicks (56 days).

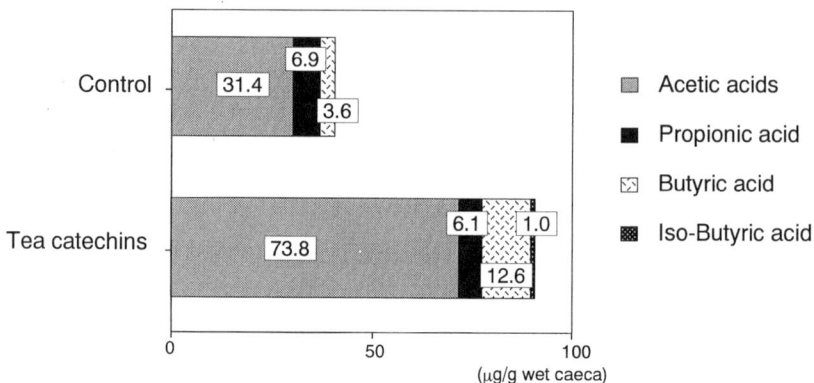

FIG. 8 Effect of tea catechin administration (0.07% of diet) on caecal volatile fatty acids of chicks (56 days).

significantly. Putrefactive products, ammonia, and ethylphenol decreased significantly and other compounds decreased not significantly (Fig. 7). Conversely, total volatile organic acids, acetic acid and butyric acid increased significantly in the catechin fed group (Fig. 8).

These results imply that catechin feeding will modulate conditions in the flora in such a way for lactic acid bacteria to proliferate relatively better than other compounds resulting in more acidic and less putrefactive products in the intestine and feces.

V. EFFECT OF TEA CATECHINS ON INTESTINAL FLORA OF PIGS

The same diet (0.07% of catechins supplemented) as above was fed to pigs for a period of two weeks (7). Results showed that tea catechin feeding markedly decreased the putrefactive products in the feces (Fig. 9). As soon as the catechin feeding was stopped, there was a sharp increase in these putrefactive products.

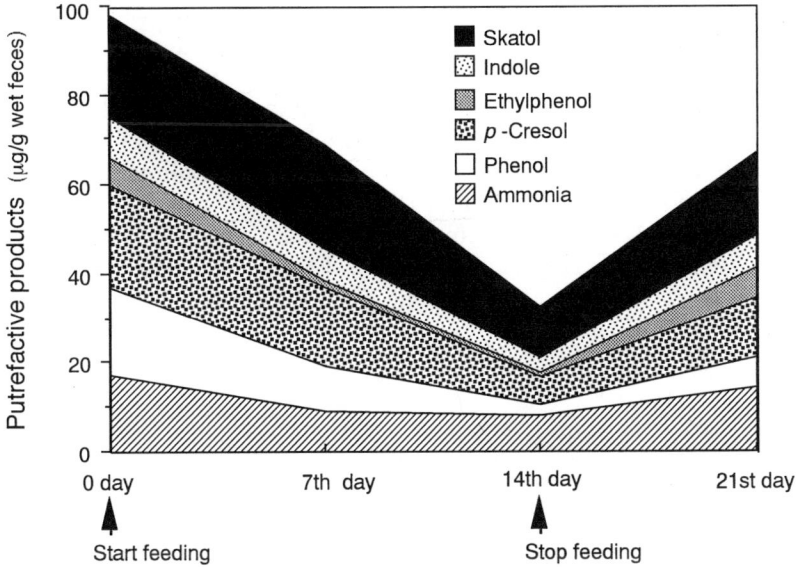

FIG. 9   Effect of tea catechin administration (0.07% of diet) on odorous compounds in pig feces.

REFERENCES

1.   N Matsumoto, F Tono-oka, A Ishigaki, K Okushio, Y Hara. The fate of (−)-epigallocatechin gallate (EGCg) in the digestive tract of rats. Proceedings of the International Symposium on Tea Science, Shizuoka, Japan, pp 253–257.

2.   K Goto, S Kanaya, T Nishikawa, H Hara, A Terada, T Ishigami, Y Hara. The influence of tea catechins on fecal flora of elderly residents in long-term care facilities. Annals of long-term care 6:43–48, 1998.

3.   Y Hara, M Honda. The Inhibition of α-amylase by tea polyphenols. Agric Biol Chem 54:1939–1945, 1990.

4.   K Goto, S Kanaya, T Ishigami, Y Hara. The effect of tea catechins on fecal conditions of elderly residents in a long-term care facility (effects of tea polyphenols on fecal conditions, Part 2). J Nutr Sci Vitaminol 45: 135–141, 1999

5.   S Kanaya, K Goto, Y. Hara, Y. Hara. The physiological effects

of tea catechins on human volunteers. Proceedings of the International Symposium on Tea Science, Shizuoka, Japan, 1991. pp 314–317.

6. A Terada, H Hara, S Nakajyo, H Ichikawa, Y Hara, K Fukai, Y Kobayashi, T Mitsuoka. Effect of supplements of tea polyphenols on the caecal flora and caecal metabolites of chicks. Microb Ecol in Health and Dis 6:3–9, 1993.

7. H Hara, N Orita, S Hatano, H Ichikawa, Y Hara, N Matsumoto, Y Kimura, A Terada, T Mitsuoka. Effect of tea polyphenols on fecal flora and fecal metabolic products of pigs. J Vet Med Sci 57:45–49, 1995.

16

The Fate of Tea Catechins After Oral Intake

Although various physiologically beneficial functions of tea catechins have been reported up until now, there is no comprehensive study that reveals how tea catechins are absorbed, metabolized, and excreted qualitatively as well as quantitatively. The compound (+)-catechin, which is a trace constituent and of the least physiological potency among tea catechins, has been examined in several reports by Griffiths et al. on the metabolic changes in animals (1) or in humans (2). After oral intake, (+)-catechin was confirmed to be absorbed and undergo methylation and conjugation in the liver and be excreted partly in the bile and mostly in the urine.

EGCg is quantitatively dominant and physiologically the most potent among tea catechins, and we traced its fate in the digestive tract of rats (3). Fifty mg of EGCg was administered orally to fasted rats; then 1, 2, 5, 8, 12, 16, and 20 hours thereafter, residual content of EGCg in the stomach, small intestine, large intestine, as well as in the feces was determined.

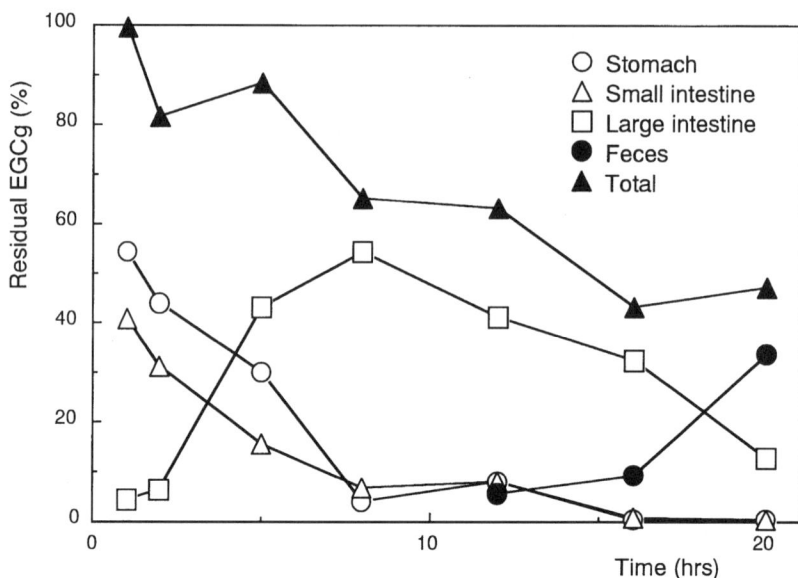

FIG. 1 Residual EGCg in different sections of the digestive tract of rats administered 50 mg of EGCg.

As shown in Fig. 1, within a few hours after administration, the EGCg in the stomach disappeared rapidly and moved into the small intestine. The amount of EGCg in the large intestine began to increase sharply as the amount in the small intestine decreased, and was at its highest around eight hours after ingestion, at which time only a trace amount remained in the other organs. EGCg appeared in the feces 12 hours after ingestion and increased gradually thereafter. In the two hours after administration, when a small amount of EGCg was already in the large intestine, about 20% of the EGCg was lost (i.e., unrecoverable). We concluded that this 20% disappearance of EGCg is equivalent to the amount absorbed into the body through the small intestinal wall. This assumption is backed up by a previous report that confirms that EGCg does not undergo any degradation in the stomach or small intestine (3). Hattori et al. showed that when galloyl catechins (EGCg, ECg) were incubated anaerobically with human feces, they succumb to extensive degradation, whereas they are stable in rats' feces (4). The latter is, however, not likely in our experiment in rats with tritiated EGCg. There seems to be certain degradation of EGCg in rat's large intestine. In the following experiments with rats, we have confirmed the absorption and existence of EGCg and other individual catechins in the portal vein (5). Forty-five minutes after administering each catechin orally, the portal blood was collected and each catechin was isolated and purified from the blood. Those purified compounds were identified as individual catechins by HPLC and LC/MS analyses. We have found by incubating catechins with methyl group donor, S-adenosyl-L-methionine, in rat liver homogenates that O-methylation occurs at 4' position of EGC or 4" position in galloyl moiety of ECg and EGCg as shown in Fig. 2 (6). After oral administration of (−)-epicatechin (EC) to rats, its metabolites and the fate of them were investigated (7). We identified 3'-O-methyl-EC, 4'-O-methyl-EC, EC-5-O-β-glucuronide and 3'-O-methyl-EC-5-O-β-glucuronide as metabolites of EC. In the urine, EC-conjugates were the major forms of EC metabolites while in plasma and bile, 3'-O-methyl-EC-conjugates seemed to be dominant (Fig. 3).

More practically in humans, C. S. Yang et al. confirmed the presence and excretion of the glucuronide and/or sulfate of individual catechins in the plasma and urine of subjects who took 1.2 gram of decaffeinated green tea extract powder (8). They identified catechins in the plasma, 1 to 4 hours after the intake of tea, predominantly in conjugated (either glucuronide or sulfate) forms and in the concentration range of 50–300 nanograms catechins/ml. The excretion of catechins in the urine was also predominantly in conjugated forms and began three hours after ingestion, then tended to level off after six hours. The cumulative amount of excreted catechins was only a few milligrams each as compared to the total amount of 235 mg catechins contained in the extract powder administered. Reviewing all the above data in addition to our unpublished results, it is thought to be very likely that tea catechins taken

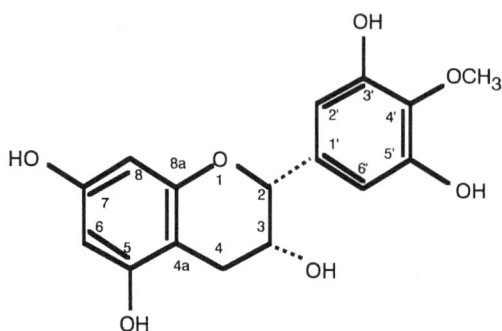

FIG. 2 Structures of methylated (−)-epigallocatechin, (−)-epicatechin gallate, and (−)-epigallocatechin gallate formed by a rat liver homogenate.

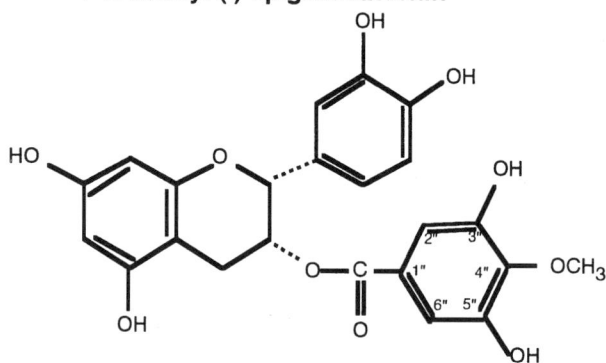

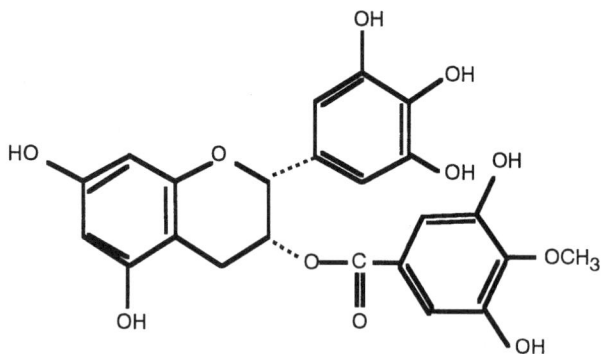

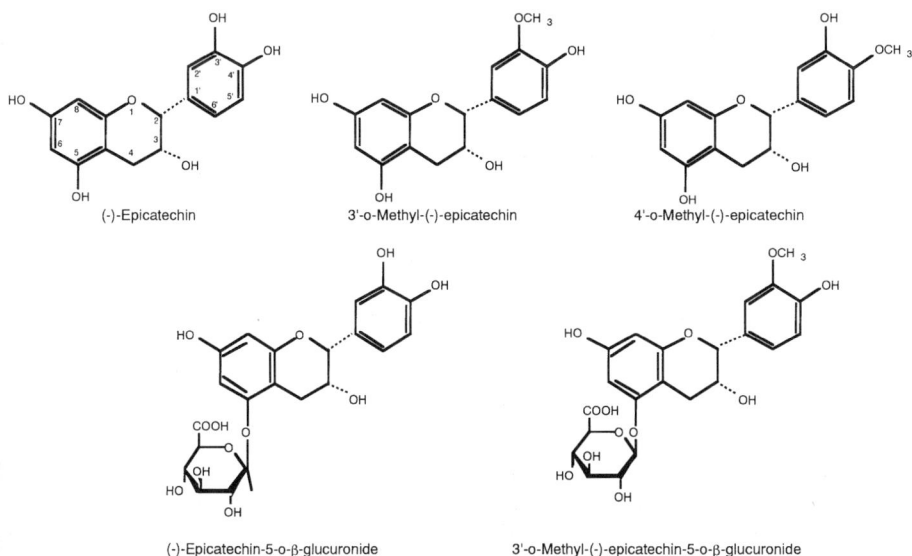

FIG. 3   Structures of (−)-epicatechin metabolites.

orally by humans will enter the small intestine and a part of
them undergo conjugation in the process of absorption into the
portal vein. In the liver, catechins undergo conjugations as
well as methylations and a part of them is excreted into the
bile, while the rest is excreted into urine. The majority of unabsorbed catechins travel to the large intestine and undergo
certain degradation, entering the feces. Detailed studies of the
distribution and elimination of tea catechins after oral intake
are yet to be made. Using animals, this could be achieved by
the use of labeled compounds. Stable, tritiated EGCg was prepared in the laboratory of Mitsui Norin Co., Ltd., in 1999, and
its fate in rats is under detailed study. (Result to be published.)

REFERENCES

1.   IC Shaw, LA Griffiths. Identification of the major biliary metab-
      olite of (+)-catechin in the rat. Xenobiotica 10:905–911, 1980.

2. M Wermeile, E Turin, LA Griffiths. Identification of the major urinary metabolites of (+)-catechin and 3-O-methyl-(+)-catechin in man. European J of Drug Metabolism and Pharmacokinetics 8:77–84, 1983.
3. N Matsumoto, F Tono-oka, A Ishigaki, K Okushio, Y Hara. The fate of (−)-epigallocatechin gallate (EGCg) in the digestive tract of rats. Proceedings of the International Symposium on Tea Science, Shizuoka, Japan, 1991.
4. MR Meselhy, N Nakamura, M Hattori. Biotransformation of (−)-epicatechin 3-O-gallate by human intestinal bacteria. Chem Pharm Bull 45:888–893, 1997.
5. K Okushio, N Matsumoto, T Kohri, M Suzuki, F Nanjo, Y Hara. Absorption of tea catechins into rat portal vein. Biol Pharm Bull 19:326–329, 1996.
6. K Okushio, M Suzuki, N Matsumoto, F Nanjo, Y Hara. Methylation of tea catechins by rat liver homogenates. Biosci Biotechnol Biochem 63:430–432, 1999.
7. K Okushio, M Suzuki, N Matsumoto, F Nanjo, Y Hara. Identification of (−)-epicatechin metabolites and their metabolic fate in the rat. Drug Metabolism and Disposition 27:309–316, 1999.
8. MJ Lee, ZY Wang, H Li, LS Chen, Y Sun, S Gobbo, DA Balantine, CS Yang. Analysis of plasma and urinary tea polyphenols in human subjects. Can Epi, Biomarkers & Prev 4:393–399, 1995.

17

Efficacy of the Health Benefits of Black Tea or Black Tea Polyphenols

I. INTRODUCTION

Although a multitude of beneficial health effects of catechins obtained from green tea have been dealt with in this book, in this context, no detailed mention has been made thus far of black tea polyphenols. Yet, the merit of theaflavins or black tea infusion was noted in several chapters (see those actions on antiflu, antibacterial, anticarious, antilipidemic, antitumorigenic, inhibition of α-amylase, angiotensin-converting enzyme, or LDL oxidizability). In this chapter, I would like to briefly discuss the complexity of study on black tea and describe several functions of black tea polyphenols.

In tea gardens around the world, shoots of the tea bush contain from 15% to over 20% (dry weight basis) of catechins. Teas grown in temperate zones such as China or Japan are made into green tea, while those grown in tropical regions such as India or Sri Lanka are processed mostly as black tea.

Mild sunshine produces less pungent (lower catechin content) and sweeter (relatively higher amino acid content) tea shoots, which are suited to the production of green tea. In the tropical tea garden, as a means perhaps for coping with the strong sun rays and more persistent external vermin, tea shoots tend to hold a greater amount of catechins in their cells, giving them potent polyphenol oxidase activity. These properties of tropical tea shoots are made more palatable when processed into black tea by oxidizing catechins rather than processing them into green tea, which would produce a beverage too pungent for our palates (see "Fermentation of Tea"). Because of the above situation, polyphenols in green tea and black tea differ in the following way: Green tea polyphenols, which are composed of four main tea catechins, are all isolated and well-defined individually, hence it is possible to determine the contribution of each to a specific action. On the other hand, black tea polyphenols, which are originally composed of four main tea catechins with more than 20% combined content, are oxidized and promiscuously form oligomers or polymers, only part of which are identified and defined; that is less than 5% unoxidized catechin residue and 1–2% theaflavins (catechin dimers of defined nature). The remainder, about 15%, is a catechin complex mixture of undefined heterogeneous polymers, termed tentatively as thearubigin. Content and nature of thearubigin fraction differs according to the different area of production and the season they were harvested. Thus, the methodology in search of the efficacy of black tea polyphenols needs to be different from that of green tea catechins. One method of research is to use theaflavins, which are peculiar and well-defined components of black tea, though the amount contained in the total black tea polyphenols is minimal and their isolation is a laborious work. Another way is to examine the effects of the whole black tea extract as well as the polyphenol fraction; though the results may be influenced by partiality of the sampled tea and so judgment may have to be reserved in attributing efficacy to all black tea polyphenols.

With the above limitations in mind, some of the studies made on black tea are examined.

II. ANTIOXIDATIVE POTENCY

Antioxidative potency of theaflavins was determined in a lipid peroxidation system (1). Erythrocyte membranes are prone to peroxidation because of their high content of polyunsaturated lipids. Peroxidation of rabbit's erythrocyte ghosts was induced by t-butylhydroperoxide (BHP) by 30 min incubation at 37°C. The presence of theaflavins and other antioxidants in this system deterred the formation of TBA reactive substance. Results in Fig. 1 show that theaflavins are more potent antioxidants than α-tocopherol. In a previous study using the same experimental system, green tea catechins showed an inhibition of

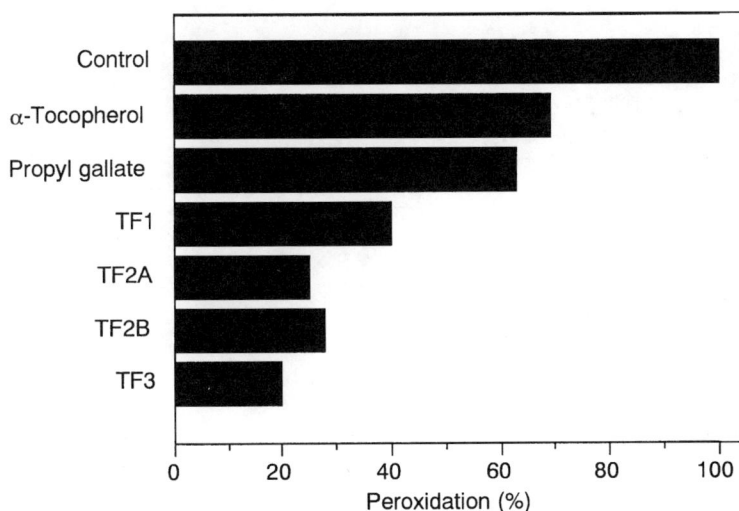

FIG. 1 Antioxidative activity of theaflavins determined by the rabbit erythrocytes ghost system. Peroxidation of erythrocyte ghost was induced by t-butylhydroperoxide (BHP). The final concentration of the antioxidants was 25 mM. The values obtained without antioxidants were used for 100% lipid peroxidation.

lipid peroxidation equal to that of α-tocopherol (2). These results indicate that the antioxidativity of theaflavins is as effective or more effective than that of α-tocopherol or epigallocatechin gallate (EGCg).

In the same way, Yoshino et al. determined the antioxidativity on lipid peroxidation of rat liver homogenates induced by BHP with theaflavins, thearubigin and infusion of black tea as well as other antioxidants (3). As shown in Table 1, the inhibition concentration (IC_{50}) of theaflavins and thearubigin was as low as that of green tea catechins with one digit lower figures than vitamin C, α-tocopherol or BHA. In this system, the lyophilized infusions of green tea and black teas showed almost identical antioxidativity.

By pulse radiolysis method, redox properties of theaflavin radicals were studied by Jovanovic et al. (4). The rate constant of the theaflavin reaction with the superoxide radical

TABLE 1 IC_{50} of Several Antioxidants on the Peroxidation of Rat Liver Homogenates Induced by BHP (t-butylhydroperoxide)

Antioxidants	IC_{50} (%, w/v)	IC_{50} (M)
GSH	1.2×10^{-2}	3.9×10^{-4}
AsA	8.6×10^{-3}	4.9×10^{-4}
dl-a-Tocopherol	5.5×10^{-3}	1.3×10^{-4}
BHT	2.2×10^{-3}	9.7×10^{-5}
(+)-Catechin	1.8×10^{-3}	6.0×10^{-5}
BHA	1.6×10^{-3}	8.9×10^{-5}
EC	1.1×10^{-3}	3.8×10^{-5}
Thearubigin (TR)	5.0×10^{-4}	—
Theaflavin (TF1)	4.9×10^{-4}	8.7×10^{-6}
Ethyl gallate	4.7×10^{-4}	2.4×10^{-5}
TF2A	4.1×10^{-4}	5.7×10^{-6}
ECg	3.8×10^{-4}	8.6×10^{-6}
EGC	2.6×10^{-4}	8.5×10^{-6}
EGCg	2.6×10^{-4}	5.6×10^{-6}

IC_{50} (M) of TR could not be calculated because of the heterogeneity and uncertainty of the molecular weight. TF2A contained a considerable amount of TF1 as an impurity.

was much higher than that of EGCg, though the reduction potential of EGCg was much lower, i.e., more likely to donate an electron, than that of theaflavin. Reactivity of vitamin E with these compounds was studied. As a result, it was postulated that theaflavin radicals, formed by the reaction of theaflavin with peroxy radicals, may potentially oxidize vitamin E, whereas on the other hand EGCg repairs vitamin E radicals.

III. INHIBITION OF MUTAGENICITY AND TUMORIGENECITY

Various heterocyclic amines have been confirmed to be mutagenic in vitro and induce cancers in animals. The inhibition of PhIP mutagenicity by theaflavins and other polyphenolic compounds has been reported (5). PhIP (2-amino-1-methyl-6-phenylimidazo[4,5-b] pyridine) is one of the heterocyclic amines prevalent in our daily life since it is produced during frying or broiling of meats and fish. The mutagenicity of PhIP in *Salmonella typhimurium* TA98 with S9 activation system was inhibited dose dependently in the presence of theaflavins as well as galloyl catechins (EGCg and ECg). The 50% inhibition concentrations of polyphenolic compounds are shown in Table 2. PhIP is a procarcinogen and activated to proximate carcinogen in the presence of P-450 enzyme contained in S9 fraction obtained from rat's liver. When theaflavins and galloyl catechins were treated with proximate carcinogen, which needs no activation by P-450, no suppression of the mutagenicity was seen in *S. typhimurium* TA98 system. Therefore, Weisburger et al. concluded that the anitimutagenic properties of these phenolic compounds may be due to their inhibition of the cytochrome P-450 enzymes.

Animal experiments were conducted by Wang et al. (6) where black tea infusion (as well as green tea infusion) was administered to mice as a sole drinking liquid while SKH-1 mice were radiated with ultraviolet B light twice a week for 31 weeks after topically initiating by DBMA. The infusion was

TABLE 2   Inhibition by Polyphenolic Compounds
of Mutagenicity Caused by 10 μM PhIP in the
Salmonella typhimurium TA98 Assay with
S9 Activation

Compound	Molecular weight	IC$_{50}$ (μM)
Catechin	290	>1000
Epicatechin	290	>1000
Epigallocatechin	306	>1000
Epicatechin gallate	442	500
Epigallocatechin gallate	458	700
Theaflavin	565	400
Theaflavin monogallate	717	180
Theaflavin digallate	869	100
Gallic acid	188	>1000
Methyl gallate	203	>1000
Tannic acid	1701	60

either 0.63% or 1.25% (tea leaves/water), the latter being just
a slightly lighter brew than our daily drinking concentration.
In the case of 1.25% infusion, the number of tumors per mouse
was inhibited as much as 93% while the size of the tumors
was markedly smaller as compared with the control group.
The intake of green tea infusion showed almost the same results as those of black tea. They observed that a decaffeinated
infusion was a little less effective than a normal brew in the
above effects. These results indicate that the risk of human
skin cancer caused by UV exposure may be reduced just by
habitual drinking of black tea.

IV. PREVENTION OF CANCER BY BLACK TEA EXTRACT OR BLACK TEA POLYPHENOLS

A study from 1985–1990 in Zutphen, the Netherlands, with
805 men aged 65–84 years, showed that dietary antioxidant
flavonoids (mostly from black tea) reduced mortality due to all

causes, with emphasis on coronary heart disease (7). This is a convincing study, but when it comes to the role of black tea in the prevention of cancer, data is limited. From the epidemiological perspective, only a couple of studies on black tea and cancer show positive data; one being a case control study on the esophagus and stomach conducted in Sweden (8) and the other being an ecological study on the uterus (9). There are a number of epidemiological studies which conclude no relationship or enhanced risk in relation to black tea drinking and cancer. It seems that more definitive studies are needed on the functions of black tea with respect to human health.

REFERENCES

1. M Shiraki, Y Hara, T Osawa, H Kumon, T Nakayama, S Kawakishi. Antioxidative and antimutagenic effects of theaflavins from black tea. Mut Res 323:29–34, 1994.
2. M Namiki, T Osawa. Antioxidants/antimutagens in foods. Basic Life Sci 39:131–142, 1986
3. K Yoshino, Y Hara, M Sano, I Tomita. Antioxidative effects of black tea theaflavins and thearubigins on lipid peroxidation of rat liver homogenates induced by *tert*-butyl hydroperoxide. Biol Pharm Bull 17:146–149, 1994
4. SV Jovanovic, Y Hara, S Steenken, MG Simic. Antioxidant potential of theaflavins. A pulse radiolysis study. J Am Chem Soc 119:5337–5343, 1997.
5. Z Apostolides, DA Balentine, ME Harbowy, Y Hara, JH Weisburger. Inhibition of PhIP mutagenicity by catechins, and by theaflavins and gallate esters. Mut Res 389:167–172, 1997.
6. ZY Wang, MT Huang, YR Lou, JG Xie, KR Reeuhl, HL Newmark, CT Ho, CS Yang, AH Conney. Inhibitory effects of black tea, green tea, decaffeinated black tea, and decaffeinated green tea on ultraviolet B light induced skin carcinogenisis in 7,12-Dimethylbenz[a]antracene-initiated SKH-1 Mice. Can Res, 54:3428–3435, 1994.
7. GL Hertog, EJM Feskens, PCH Hollman, MB Katan, D Kromhout. Dietary antioxidant flavonoids and risk of coronary heart disease. The Zutphen elderly study. Lancet 342:1007–1011, 1993.

8. LE Hansson, O Nyren, R Bergstrom, A Wolk, A Lindgren, J Baron, HO Adam. Diet and risk of gastric cancer. A population-based case-control study in Sweden. Int J Cancer 55:181–189, 1993.
9. P Stocks. Cancer mortality in relation to national consumption of cigarettes, solid fuel, tea, and coffee. Br J Cancer 24:215–225, 1970.

18

Toxicology

I. INTRODUCTION

Tea catechins are major components in green tea that have and are still being consumed abundantly by tea drinkers. Suppose 2 g of green tea (an ordinary amount in a tea bag) is brewed by hot water in a 150 cc cup, an average 80 mg of catechins are extracted in a brew. Some prefer a more pungent brew of 100 mg/cup and others prefer a lighter one of 50 mg/cup. In various epidemiological studies, heavy tea drinkers are reported to consume more than 10 cups a day. This means they are habitually taking almost 1 g of tea catechins a day. In one such study in Japan by Imai and Nakachi, where 1371 men over 40 years of age were surveyed for 5 years, 23% of them had been drinking more than 10 cups a day. Those heavy tea drinkers showed decreased serum concentration of total cholesterol, LDL cholesterol, triglycerides, and an increased proportion of HDL cholesterol as compared with the less avid drinkers (1). Even though the intake of 1 g of catechins a day seems very heavy, it may be that there is some amelioration of any possible ill effects by the interaction of catechins with various other components contained in the tea beverage. Thus, when utilizing tea catechin powders for wider consumption, in capsules, tablets or in ordinary foodstuff as fortified foods, it is necessary to confirm the safety of catechin powders per se.

II. ACUTE TOXICITY TEST

Tea catechin samples were administered orally or intraperitoneally to seven-week-old male ICR mice (10 mice per dose level). In order to determine the LD_{50} (50% lethal dose) of these tea polyphenol samples, the death rate of the animals was observed for a period of five days after the sample administration. Results are shown in Table 1. By oral intake, EGCg, the pure compound, has an LD_{50} of more than 1 gram/kg body weight. Polyphenons™ (mixture of catechins) have an even higher LD_{50}, suggesting extremely low toxicity of these powders. Take the widely utilized Polyphenon 60™ (catechin content > 60%) for instance, which has an LD_{50} of 2,856 mg/kg. This dose is interpreted in human terms as 143 g/50 kg body weight of Polyphenon 60™, which is equivalent to more than 1,000 cups worth of tea catechins at one time. Thus, it is certain that there will not practically be any acute, lethal toxicity by oral intake of tea catechins.

TABLE 1   Acute Toxicity of Tea Catechins

Tea Catechins	LD_{50} (Confidence limits) mg/kg		
	p.o.	i.p.	i.v.
EGCg	1390 (1248–1647)	150 (134–168)	195 (179–213)
Polyphenon 100	2142 (1977–2320)	166 (153–182)	
Polyphenon 60	2856 (2509–3252)	186 (168–207)	
Polyphenon 30	4647 (4378–4933)	240 (221–262)	
Polyphenon G	5576 (5253–5918)	232 (208–258)	232 (208–258)

Animals: ICR strain mice ♂ 7 weeks of age
Method of calculation: Van der Waerden

III. CHRONIC TOXICITY

In order to confirm the safety of tea catechin intake on a life time basis, rats were fed catechins in the diet for a long period of time and various parameters were measured and compared with those of the control group (2). Over a period of six months, SD rats of 10 males and 10 females, five weeks old, were fed a diet with the addition of 0.5, 1.0, and 2.0% of Polyphenon 70S™, which contains more than 70% catechins. Addition of 2.0% for a period of six months is almost equivalent to 100 cups worth of catechin intake every day for nearly a quarter of a lifespan for humans. Control groups of both sexes received no catechins. After six months feeding, rats of these four groups were euthanized. Here, the group of 2% diet group was compared with the control group. Changes in body weight and food intake are shown in Fig. 1 and Fig. 2 respectively. As is apparent from the figures, there were no significant differences in body weight or food intake between catechin and control groups. The weight of representative organs was measured, and relatively compared with those of the control's as shown in Fig. 3. Significant weight gain of the liver in both sexes and significant weight loss of the ovarium in female and

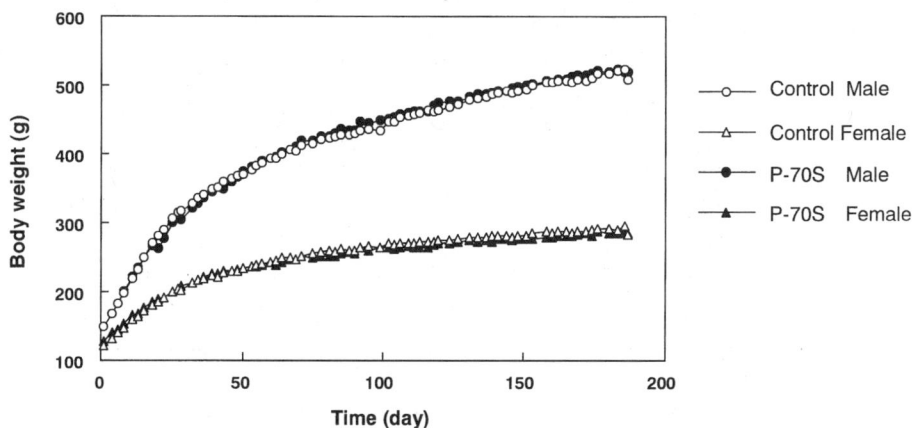

FIG. 1   Changes in body weight (SD rats).

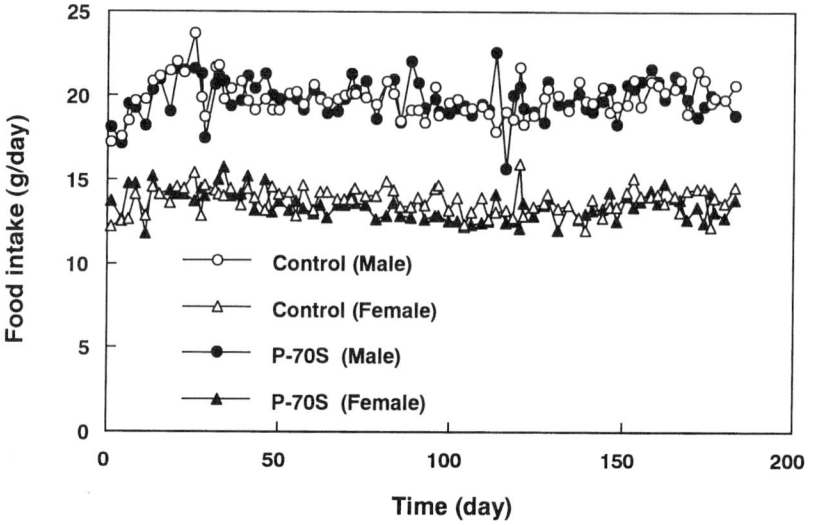

FIG. 2   Changes in food intake (SD rats).

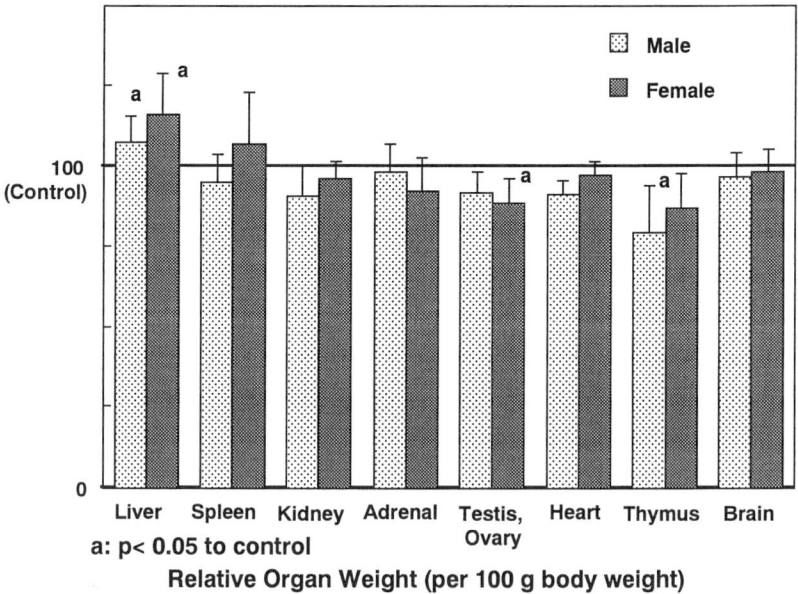

FIG. 3   Relative weight of organs. (SD rats: 2% P-70S in the diet for 6 mo.)

TABLE 2 Hematological and Biological Data

		Male		Female	
		Control	Polyphenon 70S	Control	Polyphenon 70S
n		10	10	10	9
Red blood cell	$10^4/mm^3$	946 ± 40	942 ± 41	832 ± 42	861 ± 30
White blood cell	$10^2/mm^3$	49 ± 14	73 ± 15[a]	36 ± 9	44 ± 15
Hematocrit	%	53 ± 2	54 ± 2	49 ± 4	51 ± 2
Hemoglobin	g/dl	16 ± 1	16 ± 1	15 ± 1	16 ± 1
Platelet	$10^4/mm^3$	76 ± 20	78 ± 6	63 ± 16	78 ± 10[a]
Total protein	g/dl	6.9 ± 0.7	7.0 ± 0.4	7.6 ± 0.4	7.6 ± 0.6
Albumin	g/dl	4.7 ± 0.4	4.9 ± 0.2	5.4 ± 0.4	5.5 ± 0.4
Albumin/globulin		2.1 ± 0.2	2.3 ± 0.2[a]	2.4 ± 0.2	2.6 ± 0.2
Urea nitrogen	mg/dl	17.1 ± 2.6	18.3 ± 1.9	21.4 ± 5.3	22.3 ± 2.4
Alkaliphosphatase	IU/l	304 ± 142	390 ± 113[a]	167 ± 31	331 ± 155[a]
GOT	IU/l	144.1 ± 21.6	118.5 ± 29.9	140.8 ± 43.3	202.3 ± 84.7
GPT	IU/l	50.0 ± 4.9	72.7 ± 32.6	65.8 ± 33.5	99 ± 40.8
Triglyceride	mg/dl	80.9 ± 44.4	65.0 ± 19.8	50.5 ± 19.1	68.3 ± 42.3
Phospholipid	mg/dl	129.8 ± 33.8	83.4 ± 19.7[a]	235.4 ± 23.0	119.8 ± 21.2[a]
Total cholesterol	mg/dl	72.4 ± 14.2	68.8 ± 7.0[a]	120.7 ± 15.5	104.8 ± 17.1[a]

[a] $p < 0.05$ to control

that of thymus in male were observed. Slight degeneration of hepatocytes was observed. Biological parameters are shown in Table 2. Noteworthy is the marked increase of alkline phosphatase and the significant decreases of phospholipid and total cholesterol in catechin fed groups. Overall, though slight degeneration was observed in the liver of catechin fed groups, there was no fibrosis or necrosis.

From these experimental data it is most certain that even a conceivably huge amount of catechin intake over a lifetime will not harm human beings. Catechin capsules have been administered for years to hundreds of outpatients who are carriers of *H. pylori* (3) or hepatitis C virus (unpublished data) under the supervision of medical doctors and the medications are showing the intended efficacy, without any ill side effects. The amount ranges from 900 mg to 1200 mg catechins/day, equivalent to 7 to 15 cups worth of catechins a day. The most conservative margin of tea catechin intake would be to say that as long as catechins are taken in a daily amount less than that contained in 20 cups of tea (1–2 g catechins a day), there will never be any toxicity for humans.

REFERENCES

1. K Imai, K Nakachi. Cross sectional study of effects of drinking green tea on cardiovascular and liver diseases. BMJ 310:693–696, 1995.
2. N Matsumoto, M Yamakawa, K Sohma, Y Hara. Repeated dose toxicity study of green tea extract in rat [in Japanese]. Jpn Pharmacol Ther 27:1701–1707, 1999.
3. M Yamada, B Murohisa, M Kitagawa, Y Takehira, K Tamakoshi, N Mizushima, T Nakamura, K Hirasawa, T Horiuchi, I Oguni, N Harada, Y Hara. Effects of tea polyphenols against *Helicobacter pylori*. In: T Shibamoto, J Terao, T Osawa ed. ACS Symposium Series 701, Functional Foods for Disease Prevention, Washington, DC: American Chemical Society, 1998, pp 217–224.

19

Practical and Industrial Applications

I. A SCHEME FOR INDUSTRIAL APPLICATION

In order to make use of tea polyphenols on a large industrial scale, three factors are essential:

1. Investigation of the physiological actions in vitro, in vivo, and/or in humans
2. Extraction of tea polyphenols on an industrial scale
3. Impregnation of commercial products with tea polyphenols and proof of the utility thereof

Fig. 1 shows a schematic example of the above points. In the previous chapters, various physiological functions, i.e., utilities, are described. They range from in vitro and animal experiments to some human intervention studies. In this chapter, the extraction method of tea catechins and the specifications according to their purity in relation to their practical usage are described.

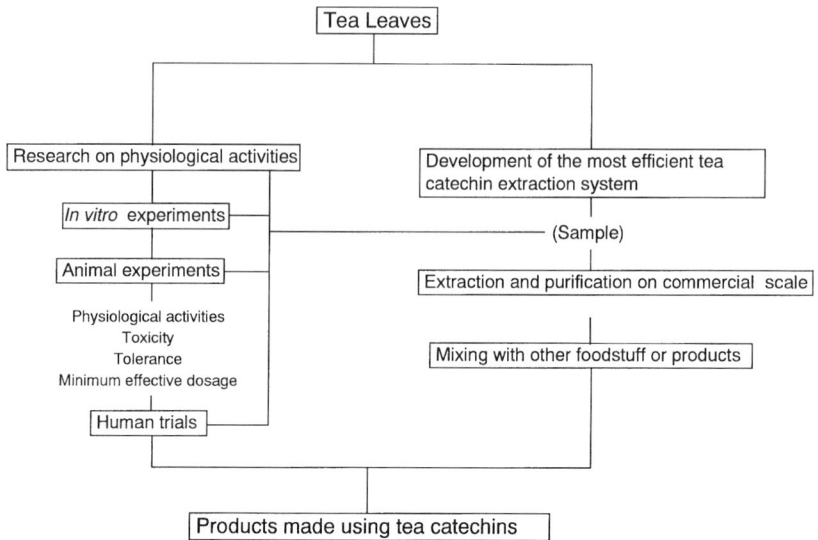

FIG. 1   Tea catechins—research and development.

II. VARIETY OF TEA CATECHIN PRODUCTS MARKETED COMMERCIALLY

Two series of green tea extracts, Polyphenons™ and Sain-catechins™, are utilized industrially for various purposes. Polyphenons are extracts of green tea, composed mainly of tea catechins, without any elements other than those of green tea. Sain-catechins are dilutions of polyphenons with large amounts of liquid, water or oils. Polyphenons with their composite and specifications are shown in Table 1.

A. Polyphenons (Fig. 2)

Polyphenon G™ has more than 25% catechin purity with less than 10% caffeine and residual chlorophyll from green tea leaves.

Polyphenon 30™ has more than 30% catechin purity with less than 10% caffeine.

TABLE 1 Composition of Catechins in Polyphenons

Tea Catechins	Polyphenon G	Polyphenon 30	Polyphenon 30S	Polyphenon 60	Polyphenon 60S	Polyphenon 70S	Polyphenon 100	Polyphenon E
(+)-Gallocatechin (+GC)	—	—	—	—	—	—	1.4	—
(−)-Epigallocatechin (EGC)	10.0	12.5	11.0	7.5	8.0	18.0	17.6	11.4
(−)-Epicatechin (EC)	1.8	3.5	2.5	8.0	4.5	7.9	5.8	9.1
(−)-Epigallocatechin gallate (EGCg)	13.5	14.5	15.0	29.0	45.5	35.0	53.9	53.4
(−)-Epicatechin gallate (ECg)	2.2	3.5	3.5	9.0	7.0	10.4	12.5	4.9
(−)-Gallocatechin gallate (GCg)						3.3		5.1
Total	27.5	34.0	32.0	63.5	65.0	73.5	91.2	83.5
Caffeine	7.0	7.0	0.5	10.0	0.5	0.5	0.5	0.5

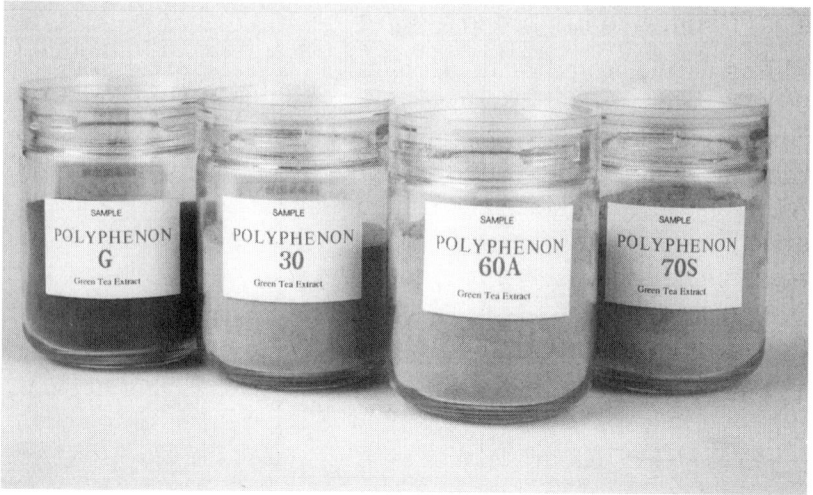

FIG. 2   Polyphenons.

Polyphenon 30S™ is a caffeine-free Polyphenon 30, with
about 30–35% catechin purity.

Polyphenon 60™ has more than 60% catechin purity with
less than 10% caffeine.

Polyphenon 60S™ is a caffeine-free Polyphenon 60, with
more than 60% catechin purity.

Polyphenon 70S™ has more than 70% catechin purity and
is caffeine-free.

Polyphenon 100™ has more than 90% catechin purity and
is caffeine-free. This variety is the same as green tea
catechin used in many of the physiological experiments
described in this book.

Polyphenon E™ is almost identical to Polyphenon 100 in
its constituents and is being produced under cGMP
standards.

B.   Sain-Catechins (Fig. 3)

Sain-catechins facilitate the use of polyphenon powders in either aqueous or oily phases. Sain-catechins are mostly used

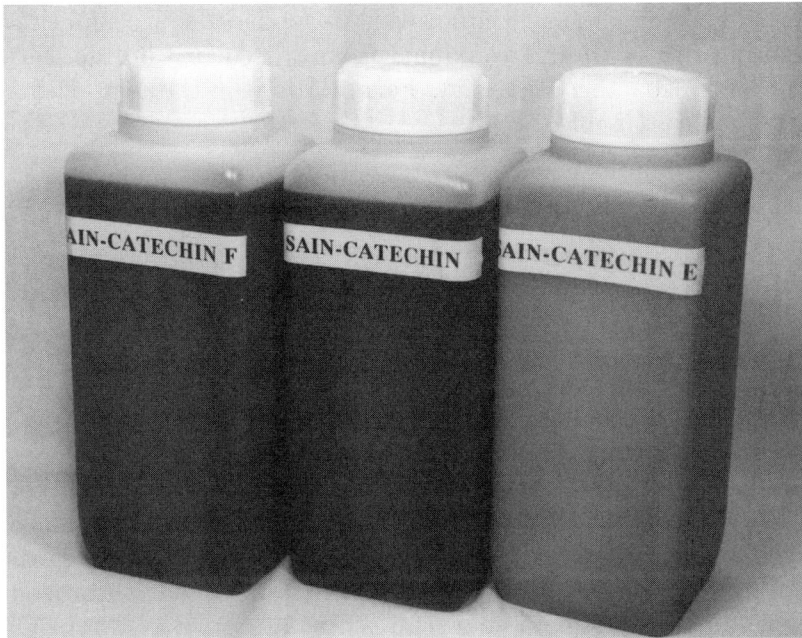

FIG. 3 Sain-catechins.

TABLE 2 Types and Packaging of Sain-Catechins

Product	Appearance	Tea catechin content	Packaging
Sain-catechin (water-soluble) (for general food products)	Brown liquid	10%	10 kg bag in box
Sain-catechin F (water-soluble) (for processed fish products)	Brown liquid	2%	10 kg bag in box
Sain-catechin E (oil-soluble) (for oil products)	Brown liquid	6%	1 kg plastic bottle in 5 kg/10 kg box

for the better preservation of various foodstuffs or cosmetics, making use of their antioxidative, antidiscoloration, deodorant, or antibacterial potency. Formulations of Sain-catechins are shown in Table 2.

III. APPLICATIONS AND PRODUCTS

A. Antioxidative Uses

1. Antioxidative Potency of Tea Catechins in Edible Oils and Their Synergism with Other Compounds

As described in Chapter 5, tea catechins have very potent effect in preventing the peroxidation of lard. Green tea catechin and EGCg, in particular, have more than 20 times more potency by weight than α-tocopherol (vitamin E) and are more than four times more potent than BHA. They also show antioxidativity in vegetable oils or even in phases of oil solubilized in water. They show synergism with vitamin E, vitamin C, and with such organic acids as citric, malic and tartaric. They are also proved to be effective in protecting the deterioration of β-carotene (vitamin A).

2. Catechin Content and Antioxidative Potency

It seems to be logical that the higher the catechin content in Polyphenons, the higher the antioxidative potency. This hypothesis was confirmed to be true in the following experiments.

Samples: Green Tea Catechin (catechin content: 91%)

Polyphenon 60™ (Catechin content: 64%)
Polyphenon 30™ (Catechin content: 34%)

These samples were mixed in a salad oil (commercial product consisting of a mixture of rape seed oil and soybean oil) in catechin concentrations of 100, 200, 500, 1000, and 2000 ppm in the oil. The oil was heated at 120°C with aeration by Rancimat method. The longer incubation time yields a better antioxidative effect. Since Polyphenon 60 has nearly twice as much catechin content as Polyphenon 30, the effect between the twofold of P-30 and P-60 is of interest. As shown in Fig. 4, at the same catechin concentrations, Polyphenon 60 shows a much better antioxidative effect than Polyphenon 30 and a little less effect than Polyphenon 100. These data indicate that one portion of Polyphenon 60 is much more antioxidative than two portions of Polyphenon 30.

3. Comparative Potency with Other Plant Polyphenols

a. Radical Scavenging Potency. Radical scavenging potency of Polyphenon 60 was compared with that of pine bark OPC and grape seed OPC in the DPPH radical trapping system. DPPH radical has specific absorbance at 517 nm. As the radical is scavenged by the antioxidant, the degree of absorbance decreases. Samples and DPPH (150 µM) were dissolved in ethyl alcohol and the decrease of absorbance at 517 nm was measured.

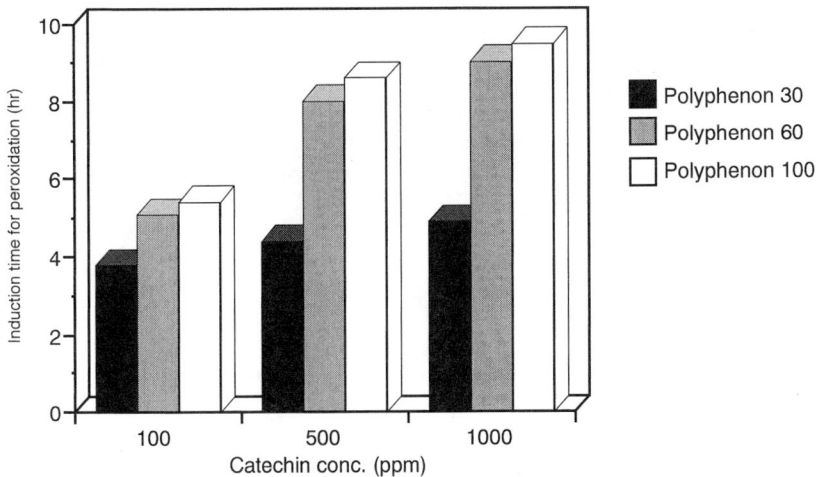

FIG. 4 Catechin content and antioxidative potency.

TABLE 3   Velocity of Scavenging Action

	Δ Abs.	Relative potency
Polyphenon 60	0.691	10.0
Pine bark OPC	0.218	3.2
Grape seed OPC	0.069	1.0

Reaction after 15 sec., sample concentration = 15 µg/ml.

1. Velocity of scavenging action.   Each sample of 15 µg/ml was mixed with DPPH and reacted for 15 seconds. As shown in the Table 3, radical scavenging velocity of Polyphenon 60 is three times higher than that of pine bark OPC and 10 times higher than that of grape seed OPC.

2. Scavenging potency per unit weight.   Each sample of 0.6 µg/ml was mixed with DPPH and reacted for 15 minutes (equilibrium). As shown in Table 4, Polyphenon 60 has the most scavenging potency by the same weight.

b. Antioxidative Test on Salad Oil.   Antioxidative potency of Polyphenon 60 was compared with those of pine bark OPC and grape seed OPC in salad oil. Samples were dissolved in commercial salad oil and underwent the Rancimat method (120°C, 20 ml/min aeration). The induction time for peroxidation was measured. Antioxidants are known to prolong the induction time. As is evident in Table 5, Polyphenon 60 showed apparent dose dependent antioxidativity at 500–1,000 ppm, whereas

TABLE 4   Scavenging Potency per Unit Weight

	Δ Abs.	Scavenged radicals per unit
Polyphenon 60	0.852	1.7
Pine bark OPC	0.675	1.4
Grape seed OPC	0.500	1.0

Reaction after 15 min (equilibrium); sample concentration = 0.6 µg/ml.

TABLE 5   Antioxidative Test on Salad Oil

Sample	Concentration (ppm)	Induction time (hr)	Relative antioxidativity
Control		3.3	1.00
Polyphenon 60	500	4.1	1.24
Polyphenon 60	1000	5.3	1.61
Pine bark OPC	1000	3.5	1.06
Pine bark OPC	2000	3.3	1.00
Grape seed OPC	1000	3.4	1.03
Grape seed OPC	2000	3.5	1.06

pine bark OPC and grape seed OPC showed no antioxidativity in this system.

4.   Product-Wise Applications in Edible Oils

Sain-catechin E mixed in edible oils (soybean oil and rape seed oil) delayed the time of peroxidation in the Rancimat test system (90°C, 20 ml/min aeration). Fig. 5 shows the time taken

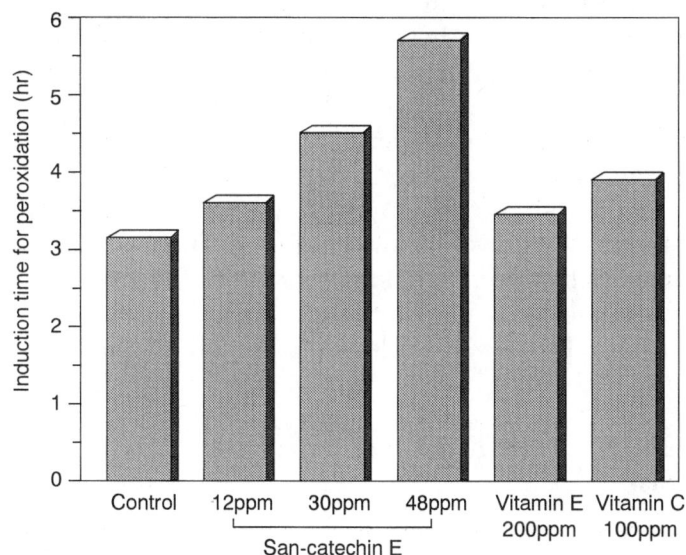

FIG. 5   Antioxidative activities of Sain-catechin E on rape seed oil.

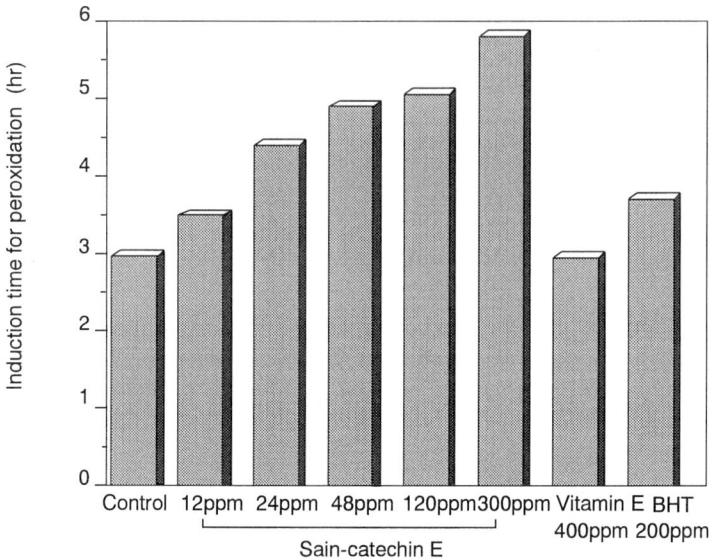

FIG. 6 Antioxidative activities of Sain-catechin E on soybean oil.

for the onset of peroxidation in oil. Sain-catechin E suppressed peroxidation of soybean oil better than vitamin E and BHT. With rape seed oil, Sain-catechin E showed better results than vitamin E or vitamin C as shown in Fig. 6. In the same way, Sain-catechin E delayed peroxidation of fish oil with 27% DHA (docosahexaenoic acid) as shown in Fig. 7. The effect of Polyphenon 60 in fish oil (27% DHA) was further confirmed by measuring the POV values as shown in Fig. 8. Thus, catechins were confirmed to be effective in suppressing the peroxidation of not only animal oils and vegetable oils but also fish oils, whereas vitamin E showed little effect in all of these instances.

5. Preservation of the Freshness of Salted or Dried Fish

Fillets of salted or dried fish on the supermarket shelves are prone to oxidative deterioration, since exposure to air under

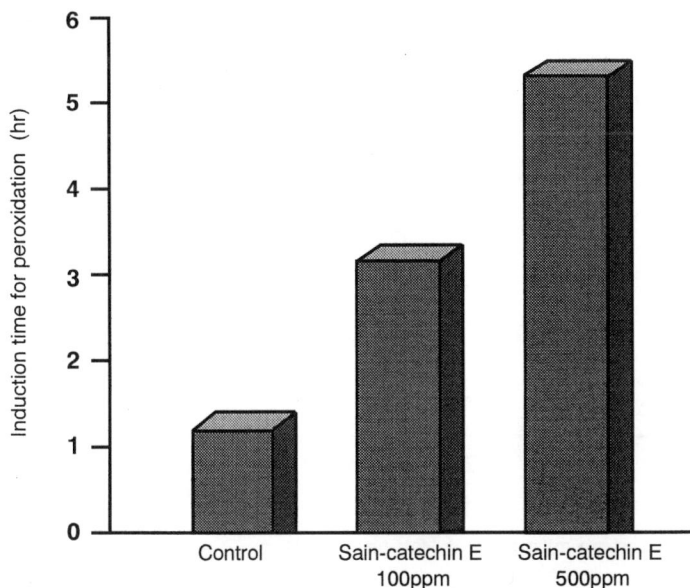

FIG. 7 Antioxidative activities of Sain-catechin E on fish oil (peroxidation of fish oil containing DHA as measured by the Rancimat method).

lights accelerates oxidation of unsaturated fatty acids in fish meat. Sain-catechin F is used widely in the Japanese fish industry to prolong the shelf life of fish fillets by immersing them in the brine with 0.5% Sain-catechin F (100 ppm catechin content in saltwater). The onset of discoloration and odor in salted salmon fillets, which usually occurs within three days, is delayed up to one week with Sain-catechin F (Fig. 9). In the same way, dried horse mackerel retained more flavor after being treated with Sain-catechin F as compared with the control (Fig. 10).

6. Suppression of Natural Food Colors

The fading of carotenoid colors is significantly suppressed by the addition of tea catechins. β-Carotene in corn oil was completely destroyed within a month under exposure to sunlight,

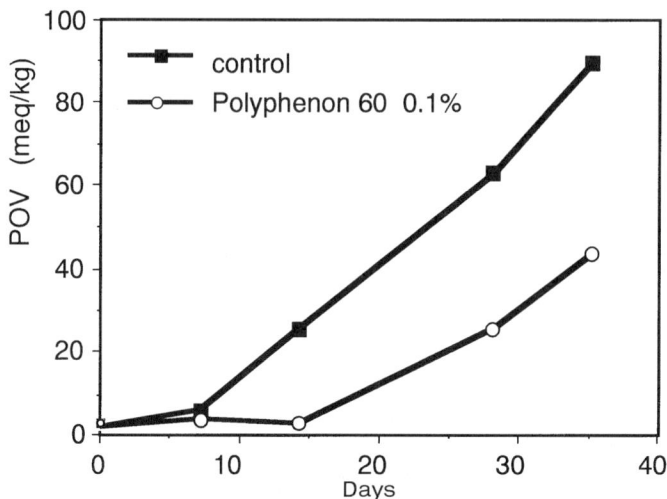

FIG. 8 Antioxidative activities of Polyphenon 60 on 27% DHA oil.

whereas the addition of 100 ppm of tea catechins (150 ppm of Polyphenon 60) kept the concentration of β-carotene unchanged (Figs. 11 and 12). It was further confirmed that tea catechins (EGCg) suppress the degradation of β-carotene at any pH range whereas the catechins commonly found in plants (+catechin; +C) have very little effect at lower pH (Fig. 13).

Tea catechins were also confirmed to suppress fading under light of natural food colors extracted from gardenia, safflower, cochineal, and monascus as well as chlorophyll and riboflavin (USP 4613672).

B. Bacteriostatic Uses

The antibacterial activity of tea polyphenols is discussed in Chapter 7 and has relevance to the soft drink industry. In acidic soft drinks there is little risk of bacterial contamination, however not all varieties are formulated acidic. Moreover, in the packaging of soft drinks, PET (polyethylence terephthal-

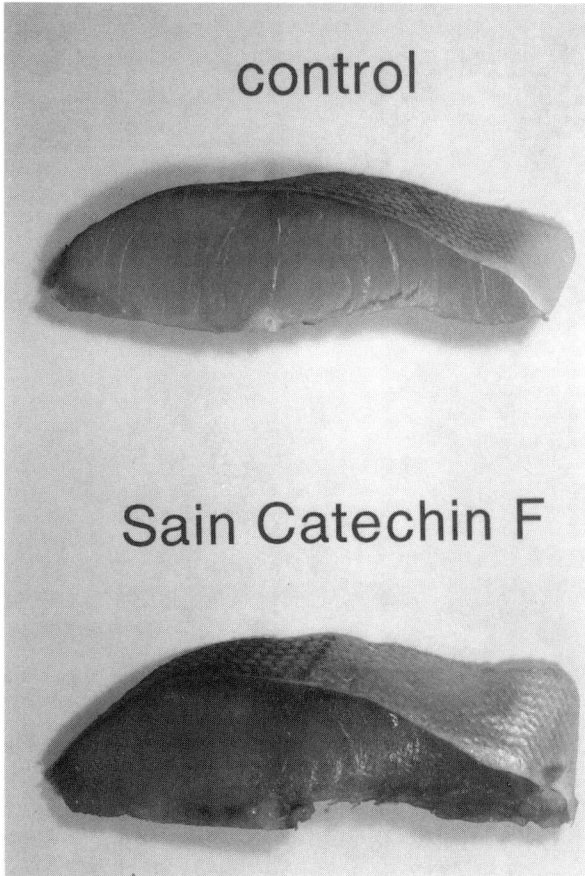

FIG. 9 Sain-catechin F.

ate) bottles are widely used by virtue of the ease of their disposal, despite the fact that they cannot withstand postfilling temperatures. Thus, soft drinks packed in PET bottles and which have a neutral pH range are not perfectly free from bacterial contamination. In most cases, heat tolerant bacteria, in particular *Bacillus* or *Clostridium,* are found in contaminated, i.e., incompletely sterilized bottles.

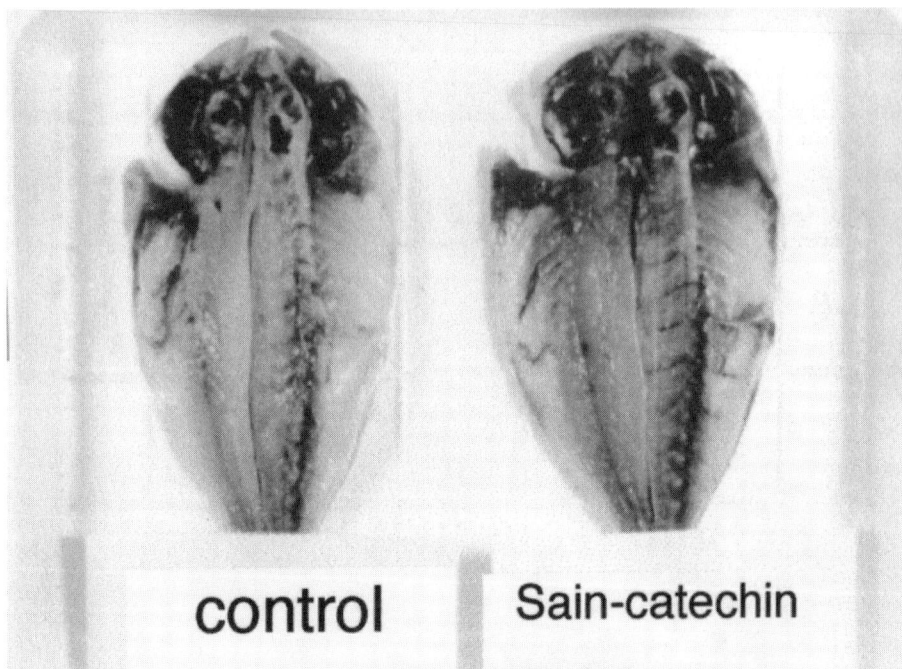

FIG. 10 Sain-catechin F as compared with the control.

The antibacterial potency of Polyphenon 30 was determined in physiological saline solution with various species of *Bacillus* and *Clostridium*. The results in Table 6 show that Polyphenon 30 has bactericidal potency below 300 ppm (catechin concentration: 100 ppm) against heat tolerant *Clostridium* and against *cereus*, *coagulans*, and *stearothermophilus* of the *Bacillus* bacterium. In the case of catechin-resistant *Bacillus*, the whole solution was heated at 90°C for 30 seconds. As a result, the bactericidal concentration of Polyphenon 30 was almost halved, as shown in the table. These results indicate that the addition of tea catechins is useful in protecting against contamination of PET bottled soft drinks of neutral pH. Several herbal soft drink brands have been fortified with tea catechins.

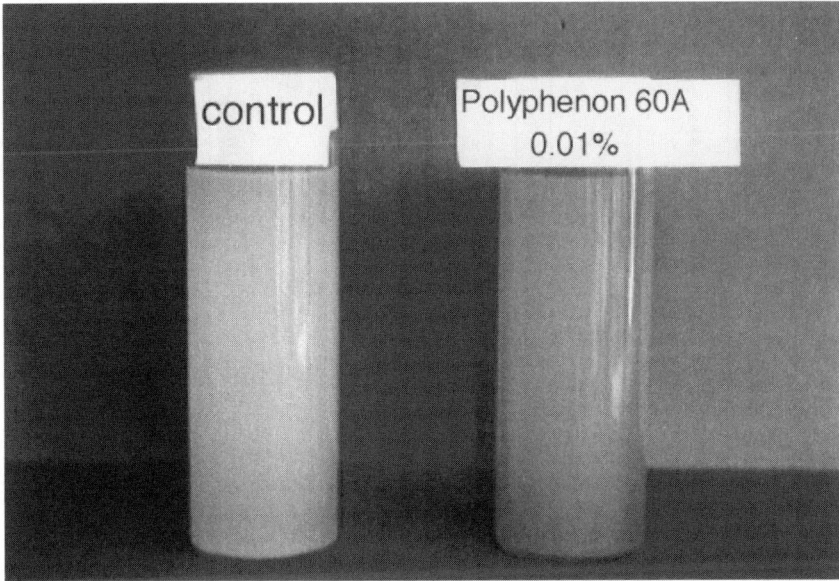

FIG. 11 Suppression of natural food colors.

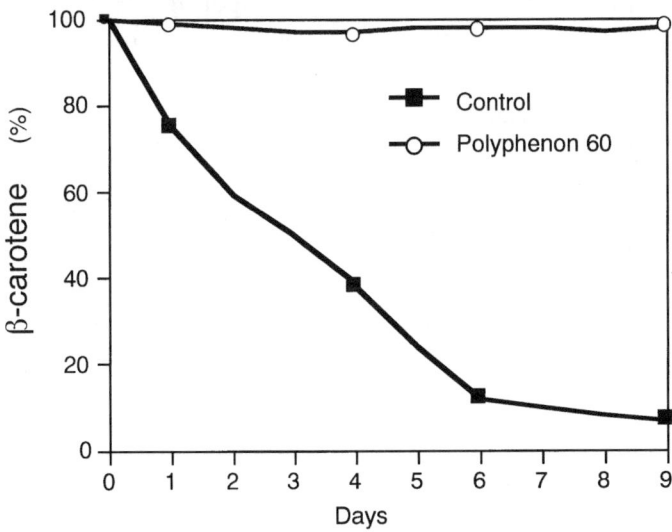

FIG. 12 The effect of Polyphenon on β-carotene fading.

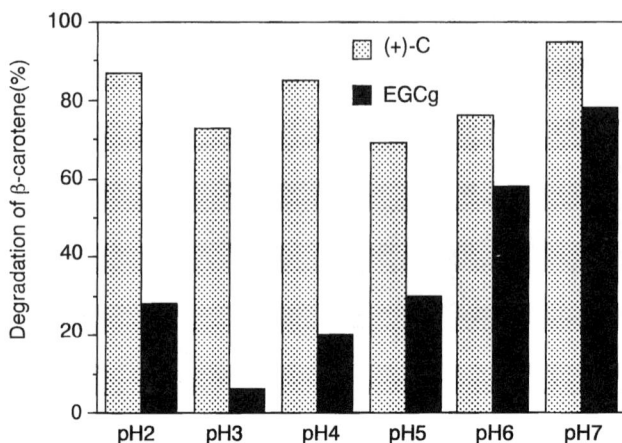

FIG. 13 The effects of pH on the protective ability of (+)-C and EGCg against β-carotene fading.

C. Deodorant Actions

1. Halistosis

Methylmercaptan (CH_3SH) is the main compound responsible for bad breath. In a flask, methylmercaptan was added to a

TABLE 6 Effect of Polyphenon 30 on Heat Resistant Bacteria (MIC of Polyphenon 30:ppm)

Heat resistant bacteria	No heat treatment	90°C 30 sec.
Bacillus subtilis	800	—
B. stearothermophilus	100	—
B. coagulans	100	—
B. cereus	200	—
B. licheniformis	600	300
B. circulans	400	200
B. polymyxa	600	300
Sporolactbacillus inulinus	100	—
Clostridium tertium	100	—
C. sporogenes	100	—
C. acetobutylicum	200	—

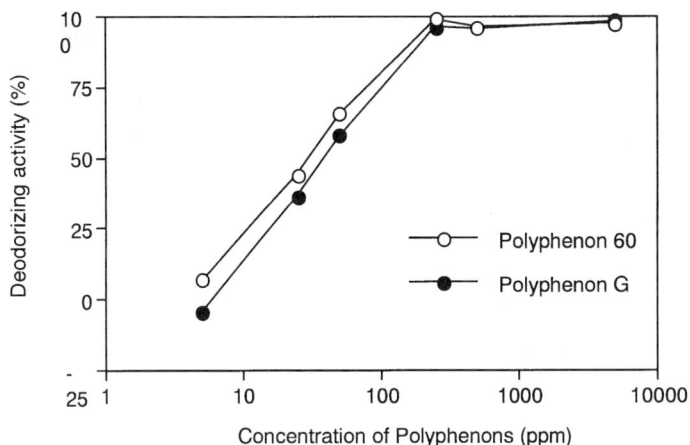

FIG. 14 The deodorizing activity of Polyphenons against methyl mercaptan (12.5 ppm) after 20 min.

buffer solution of polyphenons (variable concentrations at pH 7.5), to make up a 12.5 ppm concentration solution. The flask was incubated at 37°C for 30 minutes and the headspace gas was analyzed by gas chromatography. As shown in Fig. 14, both Polyphenon 60 and Polyphenon G, at 500 ppm concentrations, completely deodorized methylmercaptan.

Polyphenons showed a potent deodorizing effect on Methylmercaptan. The concentration of methylmercaptan normally present and noticed in the breath is below 1 ppm, as shown in Table 7. The concentration of 12.5 ppm in the above experiment is extremely high. In commercial products,

TABLE 7 Concentration of CH_3SH and Sensory Evaluation

Concentration of CH_3SH (ppm)	Degree of odor	Evaluation
less than 0.2	−	No breath odor was noticed
0.2 ~ 0.29	±	Slight odor was noticed at times
0.3 ~ 0.49	+	Breath odor was noticed
more than 0.5	+ +	Strong breath odor was noticed

for example, mouthwash or chewing gum, the addition of less than 100 ppm of polyphenons will work as a deodorizer against bad breath. At the same time, these data well explain the wisdom of the Japanese custom of drinking a cup of green tea after a meal, since the catechin concentration in a daily cup is about 500–1000 ppm, which is more than enough to deodorize the mouth and breath.

2. Meat Products

Hamburgers, particularly those made from cheap meats, develop peculiar and unsavory meat odors when cooked. Polyphenons were mixed in the minced meat and the odor of the hamburger was assessed by sensory evaluation method. As shown in Fig. 15, 0.2% Polyphenon RB added to minced meat effectively suppressed the offensive odor of the hamburger (Polyphenon RB is an extract of polyphenolic fraction of black tea).

3. Deodorizing Effect on Stools

The effects of polyphenons on stools is discussed in Chapter 15.

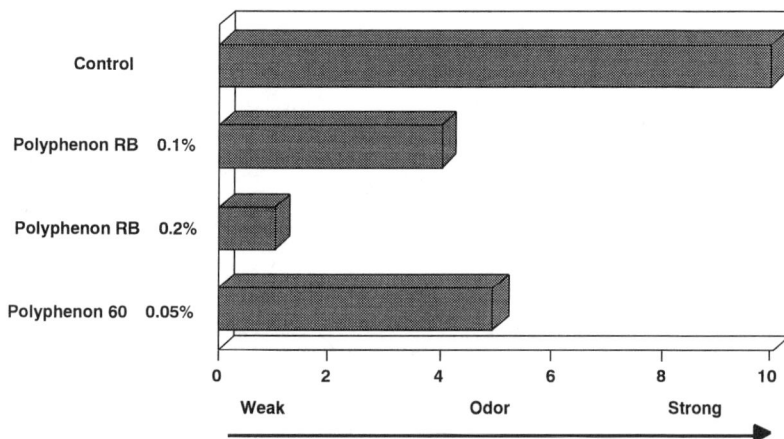

FIG. 15 The deodorizing effect of polyphenons in hamburger meat.

4. Trapping of Formaldehyde by Tea Catechins

Sick house syndrome is a serious air quality problem in homes and buildings; of which formaldehyde is recognized as being a major culprit. People develop symptoms of illness such as headaches, watery eyes, nausea, skin disorders, and fatigue when there is a buildup of formaldehyde vapor, particularly in tightly sealed houses. Building materials such as wood, plywood, or wallpaper are made with or fixed by glues in which formaldehyde is an essential component. Since plant tannins are known to react with formaldehyde, we tested the possibility that tea catechins might be able to trap the formaldehyde that is released from the glue into the air.

First, in a small glass tube with a buffer solution, 5 ppm of formaldehyde and 300 ppm of tea catechin or other tannic compounds of the same concentration were dissolved. After 15 minutes at room temperature, the solution was sampled and analyzed by high-performance liquid chromatography (HPLC). As shown in the Table 8, green tea catechins trapped almost all formaldehyde, leaving just a trace of it in the solution, whereas plant tannins were ineffective in capturing formaldehyde. Tea catechins react with formaldehyde and form an involatile compound.

Second tea catechins were impregnated into a filter in the same way as with catechin air filter (see Section E, below) and a patch of this filter was placed in a desiccator filled with a certain concentration of formaldehyde vapor. After 24 hours, the amount of formaldehyde absorbed to the filter was deter-

TABLE 8 Reactivity of Plant Tannin
Polyphenols with Formaldehyde

	Diminution rate of formaldehyde (%)
Green tea extract	97.81
Black tea extract	87.71
Quebracho extract	24.29
Mimosa extract	19.44
Chestnut extract	9.98

mined. As shown in Fig. 16, tea catechin filter absorbed form-aldehyde to a greater extent than the normal filter. The form-aldehyde was then removed from the desiccator and the formaldehyde adsorbed filters were left for another 24 hours, after which time the amount of formaldehyde released was determined. As is evident in the figure, there was only a small amount of reliberation of formaldehyde from tea catechin fil-ter. In the case of the filter without tea catechin, less formalde-hyde was adsorbed and this same amount of formaldehyde was released from the filter. Thus, cleaner air is expected with tea catechin filter.

Third, tea catechins were applied to plywood and the amount of formaldehyde adsorbed by the plywood chip was measured in the desiccator. As is shown in Fig. 17, the more catechins that were applied, the more the amount of formalde-hyde adsorbed.

Thus, since the alleviation of sick house syndrome by tea

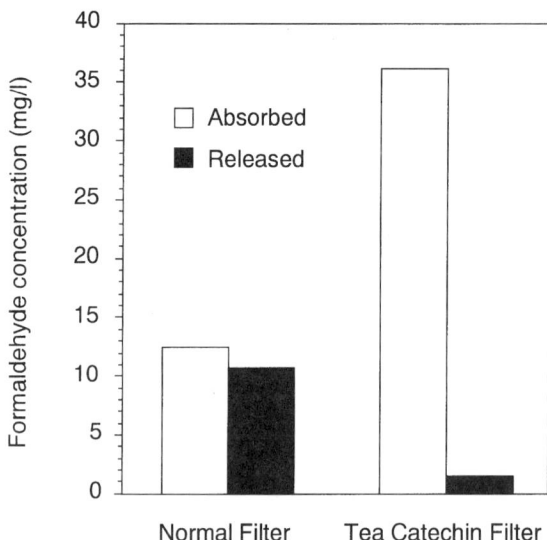

FIG. 16 The absorption of formaldehyde by a tea catechin impregnated filter.

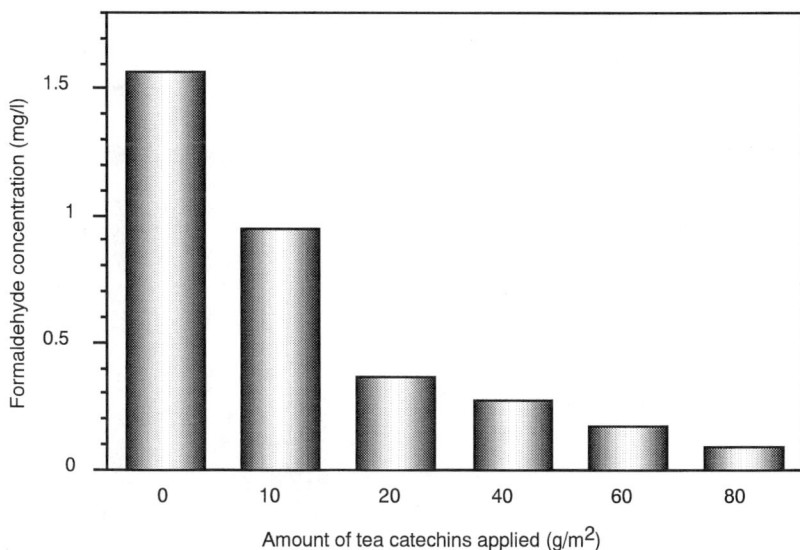

FIG. 17 Liberated formaldehyde after adsorption to plywood.

catechins is a very likely possibility, economic feasibility and practical applications of tea catechins are under study.

IV. EXAMPLES OF COMMERCIAL PRODUCTS WITH POLYPHENONS

A. Catechin 100 (Fig. 18)

For easy consumption, Polyphenon 70S is produced in a capsule form of 100 mg of catechins per capsule. This capsule is marketed under the name Catechin 100™. Catechins exert a multitude of beneficial effects in the body from the time of their oral intake to the time when they are excreted. In the oral cavity, catechins prevent various oral-airway infectious microbes as well as the influenza virus. Catechins also suppress not only the growth of carious bacteria but the formation of dental plaque.

Esophageal and stomach cancers are likely to be less

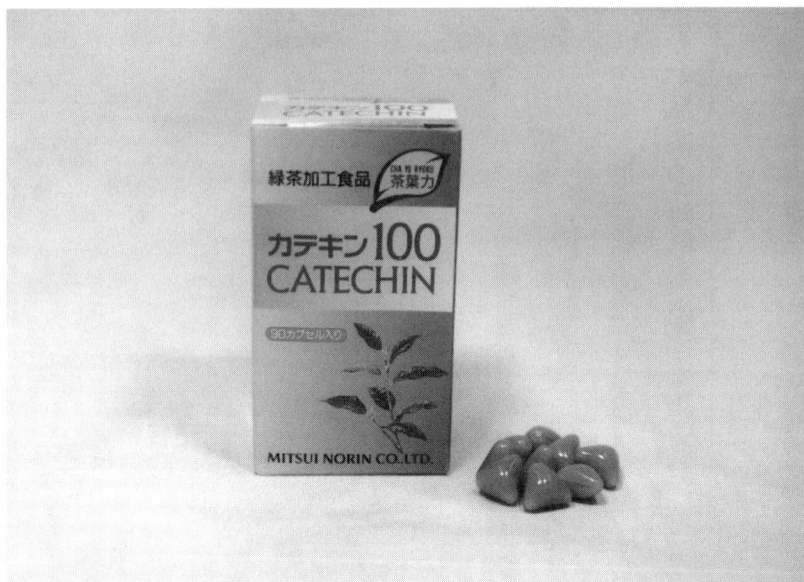

FIG. 18 Catechin 100.

among heavy tea drinkers who ingest a lot of catechins. After the intake of seven capsules of Catechin 100 every day for a month, out of 34 people who were infected with *Helicobacter pylori,* six people were proved to be free from the bacteria. *H. pylori* lives in the mucous membrane of the stomach and causes atrophic ulcer and may ultimately cause stomach cancer. In the small intestine, catechins inhibit such digestive enzymes as α-amylase and sucrase, thus preventing the over ingestion of saccharide. Catechins were also proved to suppress the ingestion of lipid by inhibiting the emulsification of lipids. Animal experiments showed, however, there will not be any malnutrition by the intake of catechins. It seems that only in the case where extra nutrients are taken, catechins work to inhibit their overingestion. Thus, Catechins are also a very safe and natural dieting agent.

Many animal experiments show the suppression of carcinogenesis by catechin intake in the small intestine and colon in particular. A trace of catechins absorbed into the vein from the small intestine is metabolized in the liver and works to suppress carcinogenesis in the liver, lung, spleen or bladder, according to the animal experiments. Catechins in the human bloodstream are likely to suppress the peroxidation of LDL cholesterol, thus lowering the chances of oxidative degradation of cardiovascular circulation systems. Most of the catechins consumed pass through the colon unabsorbed and are excreted. Catechins were proved to exert very favorable effects on the intestinal flora, increasing lactic acid bacteria and decreasing putrefactive bacteria. Very healthy bowel conditions were confirmed in humans by the administration of 3–9 capsules of Catechin 100 daily for several weeks. Various similar tea catechin capsules are sold in the U.S. health care market.

B. Catechin ACE™ (Fig. 19)

Though tea catechins work miraculously for the benefit of human health, in the endeavor to fortify the beneficial effects, other desirable components may be included in catechin ex-

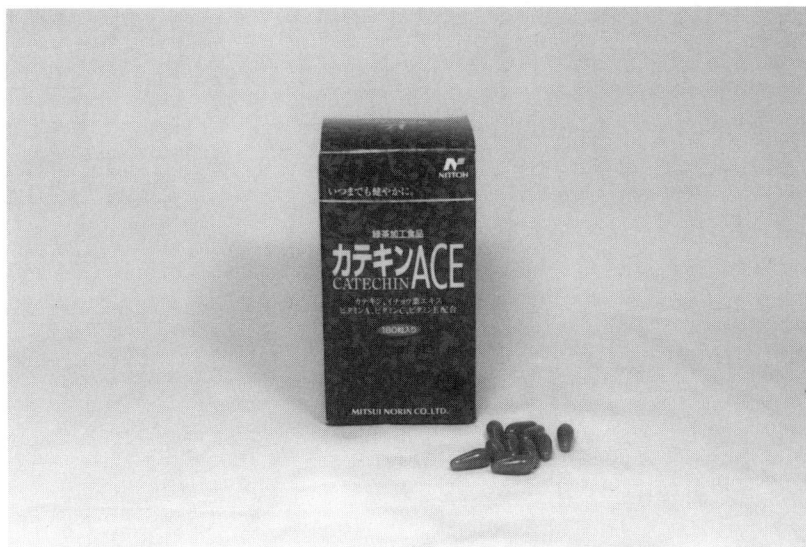

FIG. 19 Catechin ACE.

tract products. One such product is Catechin ACE in capsule form. Catechin ACE contains, in addition to 50 mg of tea catechins, 10 mg of gingko biloba extract, 200 I.U. of vitamin A, 20 mg of vitamin C and 10 mg of vitamin E. Gingko biloba extract is known to facilitate the blood circulation. Vitamin A, E, C are the most representative antioxidant components in vegetables and fruits and they each work synergistically with tea catechins to enhance antioxidativity. One capsule exerts SOD-like activity of 28,000 I.U. For those who are under oxidative stress and are prone to vascular disorders, 6–12 capsules a day are recommended.

C. Catechin 100 Plus Oligo™ (Fig. 20)

Very favorable modulation of intestinal flora by tea catechin was discussed in Chapter 15. In order to further enhance the bowel modulating actions of tea catechins, galacto-oligosaccharide was formulated with tea catechins to make Catechin 100 plus Oligo, in tablet form. Galacto-oligosaccharide is known to be a good nutrient for bifidobacteria in the intestine

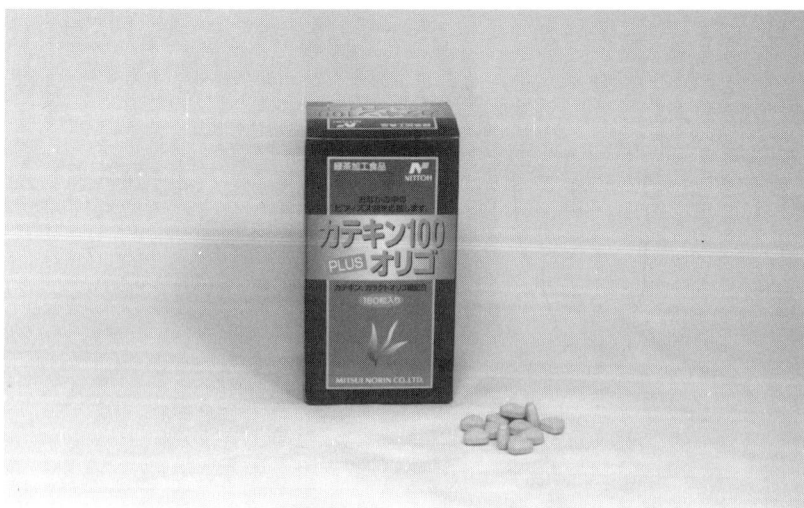

FIG. 20   Catechin 100 plus Oligo.

and to improve the condition of the bowel. Tea catechins work to inhibit the growth of putrefactive bacteria and do not interfere with bifidobacteria, thus resulting in a decrease of putrefactive bacteria and an increase of bifidobacteria or lactobacillus bacteria. In this way, the combination of tea catechins with galacto-oligosaccharide is the most ideal combination for improved health of our bowel. One tablet contains 50 mg of tea catechins and 40 mg of galacto-oligosaccharide. Daily intake of 6–9 tablets is recommended.

D. Bottled Health Drinks: β-Catechin (Fig. 21)

Tea catechins are mixed with β-carotene and various other herbal extracts to enhance the scavenging actions against oxygen radicals. This concentrated mixture is contained in a small 50 ml bottle; it is a potent health drink that can be consumed daily.

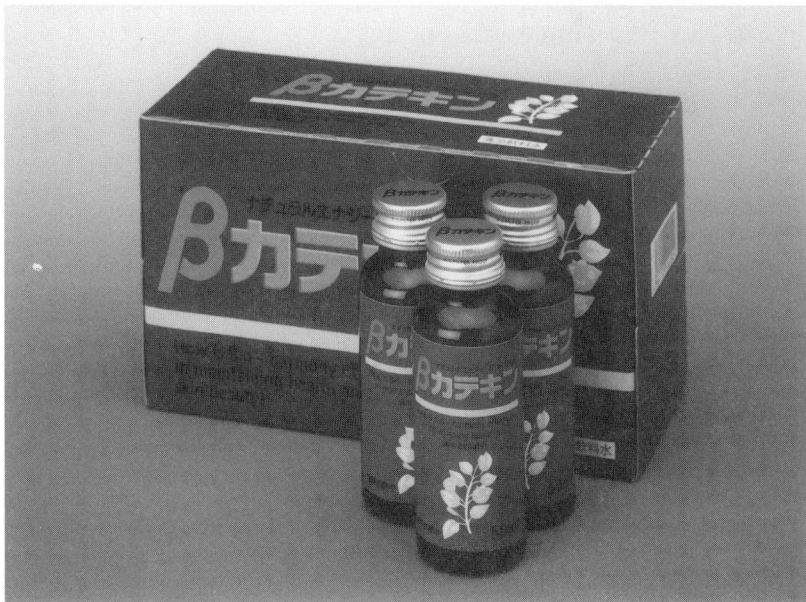

FIG. 21 Bottled health drinks.

E.   Antiflu Air Purifier (Fig. 22)

The remarkable effect of tea polyphenols in preventing the infection of influenza virus was utilized on the Catechin Air Filter. The air purifier with catechin filter was developed with the collaborative R&D of National/Panasonic and Mitsui Norin Co. Tea catechin (P-60) was impregnated in the air purifying filter by way of a special technique. The air purifier equipped with the catechin filter was proved to reduce the number of viruses sprayed on the filter from 200,000 to less than 10 in about six hours of ventilation, whereas on the filter not impregnated with catechin 170,000 viruses were counted. This was proved with the coxackie virus, which is much smaller and more resistant than the influenza virus. The catechin filter is fitted together with a charcoal filter and electrostatic filter to the air purifier. The antiviral effect of the filter is guaranteed for a year of ventilation (8 hours/day). The filter is exchangeable and a new one can be fitted when the effectiveness wears off. Several patents have been filed relative to the antiflu property of catechins and accessories that employ this property.

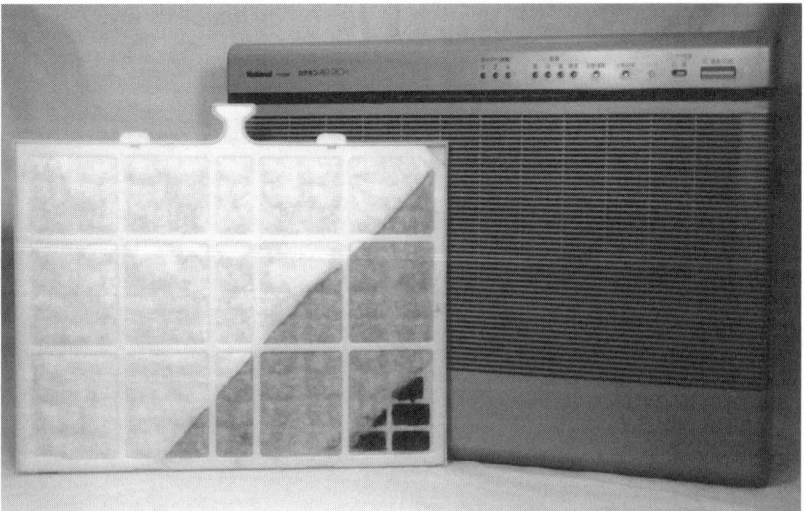

FIG. 22   Antiflu air purifier.

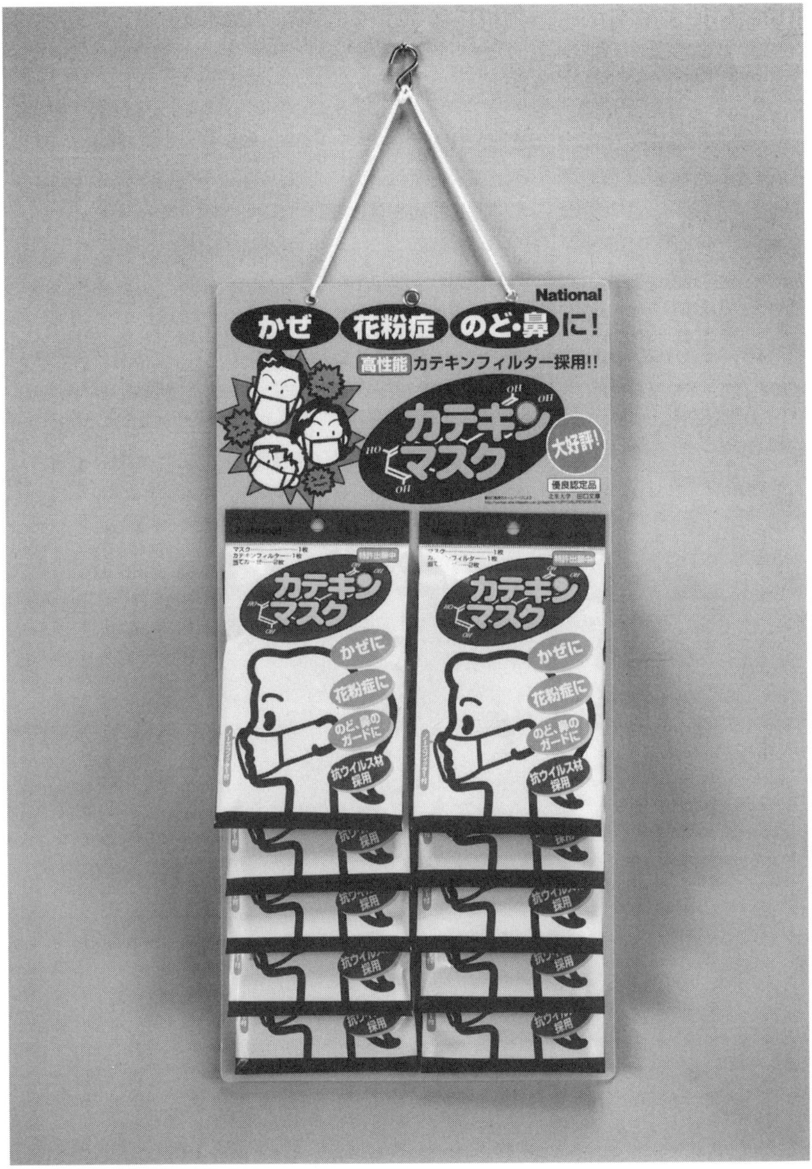
National
かぜ
花粉症
のど・鼻
に!
高性能
カテキンフィルター採用!!
カテキン
マスク
大好評!
優良認定品
かぜに
花粉症に
のど、鼻の
ガードに
抗ウイルス材
採用

FIG. 23 Antiflu masks.

F. Antiflu Mask (Fig. 23)

A small piece of catechin air filter as manufactured above was fitted in a facial mask. Wearing this mask gives some protection from airborne contamination by viruses. Use of this catechin mask is recommended particularly at times when influenza is rampant, especially for older people when they go out in cold weather, since they are more susceptible.

G. Catechin Candy (Fig. 24)

Anticipating the same antiflu effect as above, candies containing catechin have entered the market. Regulations do not allow claims concerning the efficacy, but this knowledge may be spread widely by word of mouth. Similarly, catechin chewing gum is under development.

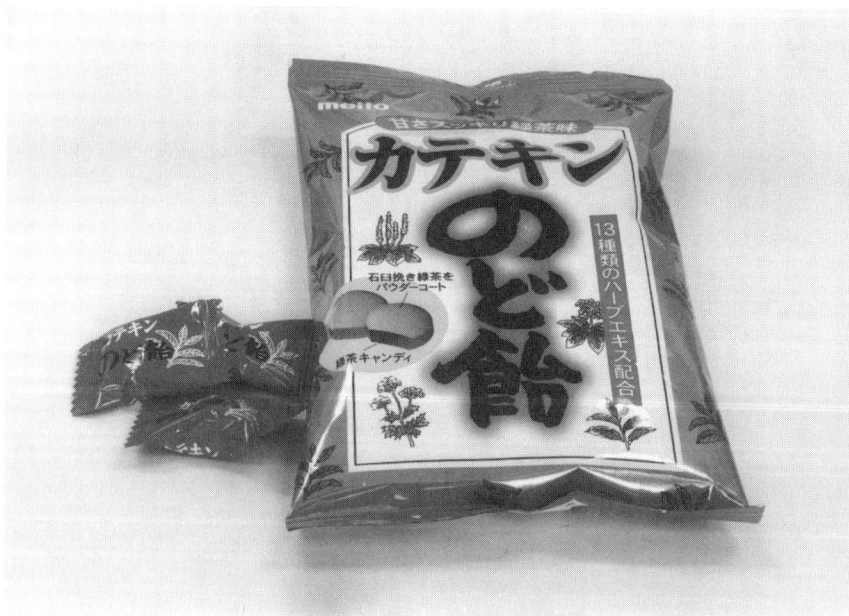

FIG. 24 Catechin candy.

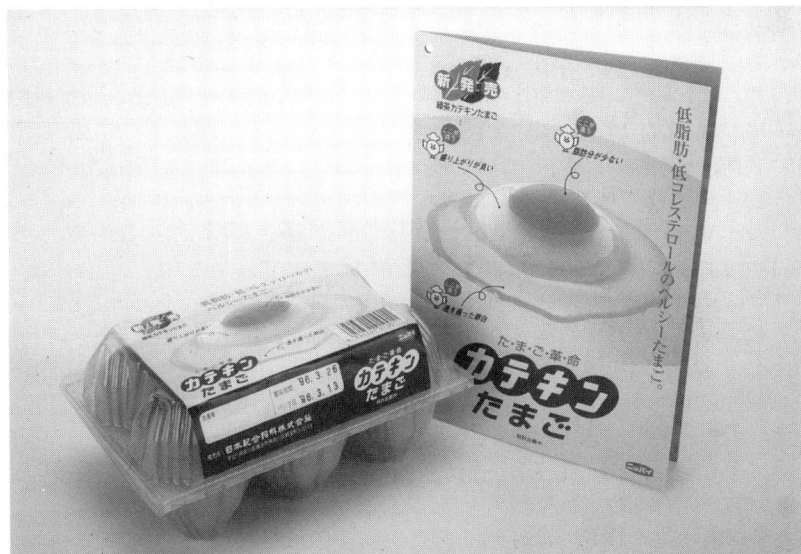

FIG. 25 Catechin eggs.

H. Catechin Eggs™ (Fig. 25)

Tea catechins mixed in the feed of laying chickens produce eggs with uniquely favorable characteristics as compared with the conventional (noncatechin) ones. As shown in Table 9, the content of total lipid and cholesterol as well as the peroxide

TABLE 9 Catechin Eggs Versus Conventional Egg

per 100g	Catechin egg	Conventional egg
Calories (Kcal)	125	162
Protein (g)	11.2	12.3
Lipid (g)	7.7	11.2
Carbohydrate (g)	1.0	0.9
Sodium (mg)	147	130
Cholesterol (mg)	321	470
Peroxide (μmol)	5.2	6.5

value in the yolk is quoted to be much lower than in conventional eggs. The Haugh unit value, which indicates the height of the thickest part of the white of an egg, is higher in the catechin egg. These factors suggest that not only does the egg have health benefits for those who eat it, but it is possible that if the egg was fertilized these health benefits may be passed on to the chick. Several other interesting features are noted in the catechin eggs. The white of the egg is totally transparent and when whipped it is pure white in color. No dark colored iron sulfide is present on the surface of the yolk when the egg is hard boiled. The production method and the particular features of this catechin egg are patented (USP 5766595). The eggs are marketed widely in Japan by Nippon Formula Feed Mfg. Co. and are gaining in popularity.

I. Cosmetics (Fig. 26)

Antioxidative potency and UV protecting functions of tea catechins (Polyphenons) are utilized in cosmetics. Cosmetic formu-

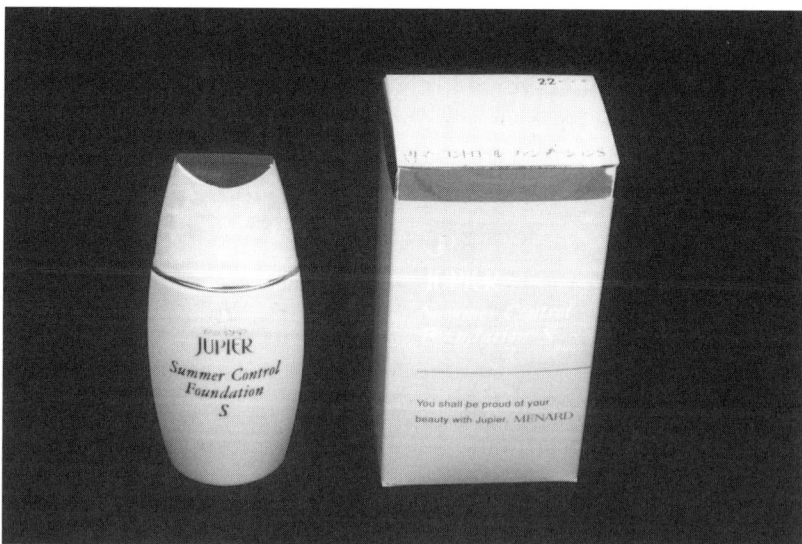

FIG. 26 Cosmetics utilizing tea catechins.

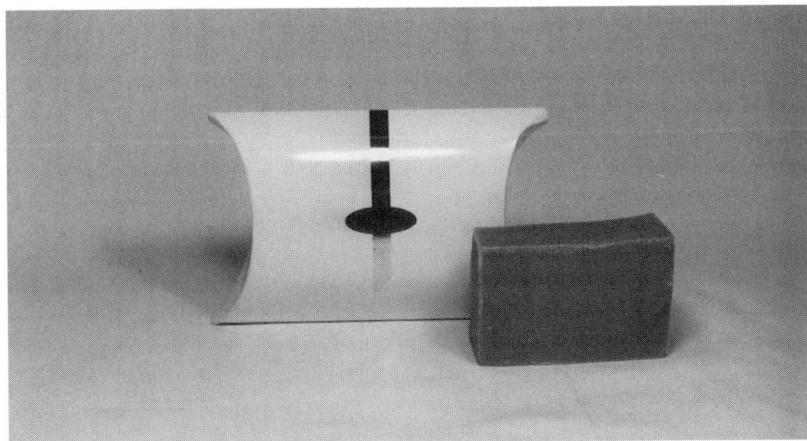

FIG. 27 Catechin soap.

las and their manufacturing processes are highly specialized techniques known only to the cosmetic manufacturers. Various products are presently on the market and there are plans for still more to be marketed.

J. Catechin Soap (Fig. 27)

Highly purified catechins are blended and made into rather crude looking square-shaped soap. Though priced high, many avid users enjoy remedial effects on skin disorders by using this soap.

K. Kitchen Deodorizer (Fig. 28)

Tea catechins are dissolved in ethanol/water and added to a hand spray. After cooking fish, a spray of this liquid removes the fishy smell. Antibacterial actions are also anticipated by using this spray on kitchen utensils.

L. Mouth Deodorizing Tablets (Fig. 29)

Taken after meals these catechin tablets can reduce odors such as that of garlic or fish. They are packaged in a convenient portable size.

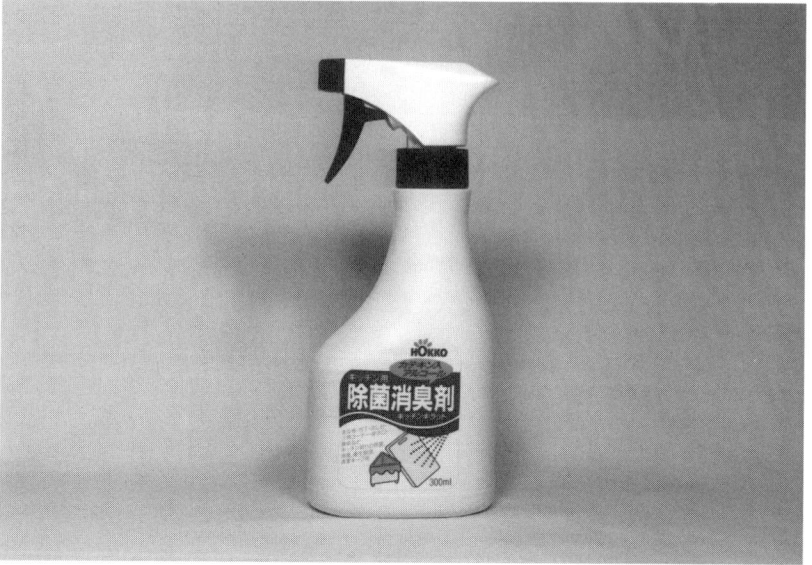

FIG. 28 Kitchen deodorizer.

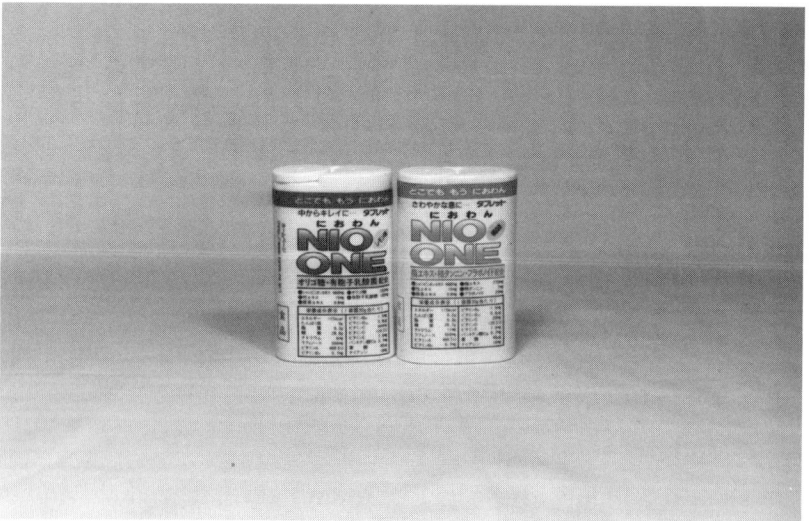

FIG. 29 Mouth deodorizing tablets.

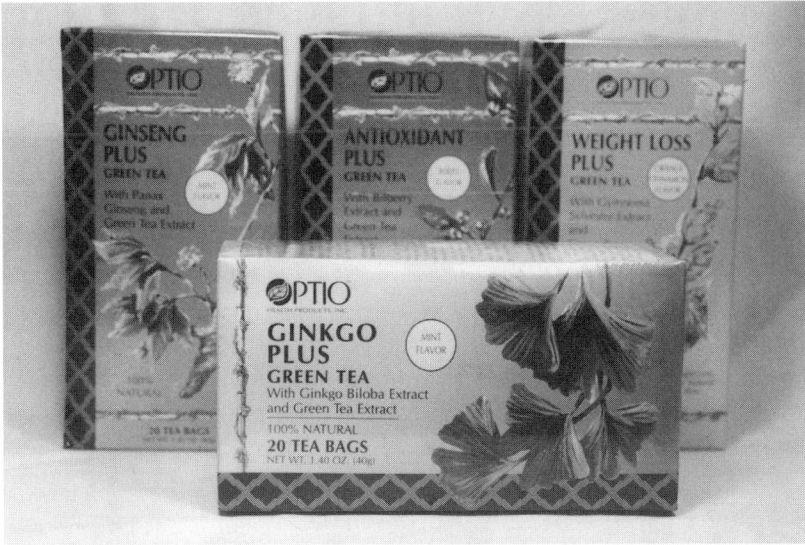

FIG. 30 Catechin-enriched tea bags.

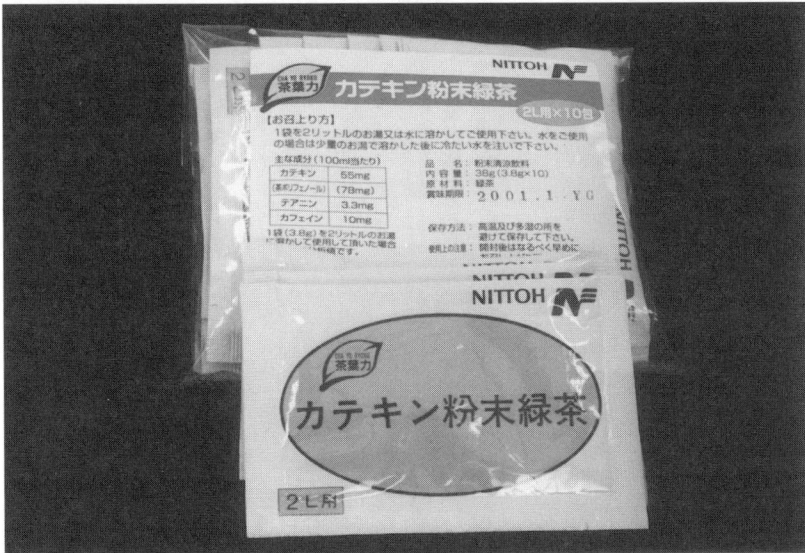

FIG. 31 Catechin Matcha.

M.   Catechin-Enriched Green Tea Bags (Fig. 30)

Powdered green tea and herbs, supplemented with Polyphenon 60, are kneaded, extruded and dried. The dried particles are put into tea bags and are being marketed in U.S.
health care stores. Gingko biloba, ginseng, gymnema, bilberry,
and several others make up the range of flavors. These teas
have been produced with the intention of making green tea
palatable to the U.S. market.

N.   Catechin Matcha (Fig. 31)

Matcha is mixed with Polyphenon and powdered milk, thereby
doubling the normal catechin content per cup and making the
taste less pungent.

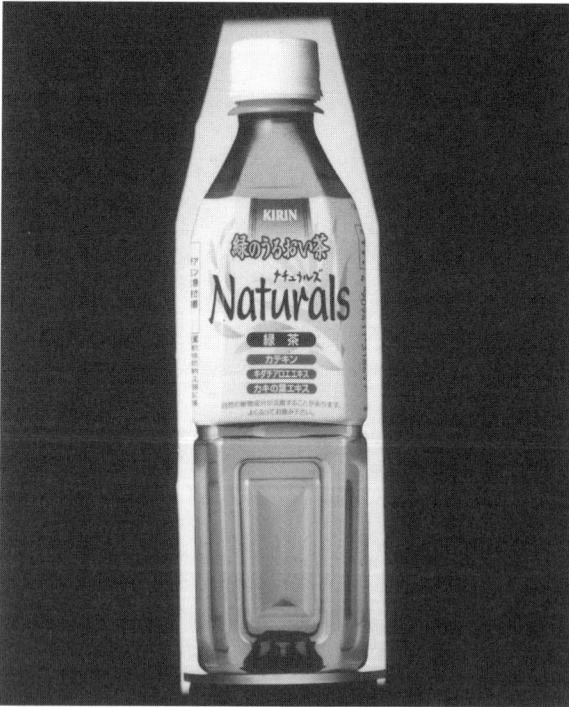

FIG. 32   Naturals, a catechin-enriched soft drink.

O. Catechin Enriched Soft Drink Naturals (Fig. 32)

This is a thirst-quenching drink made from a mix of tea catechins and other natural ingredients (500 ml PET bottle).

P. Slug and Snail Spray (Fig. 33)

This is a safe, natural spray containing tea catechin, which
exterminates slugs and snails.

Q. Pet Foods (Fig. 34)

Tea catechins were mixed in pet foods to promote good health,
and to reduce fecal odor and caries in animals.

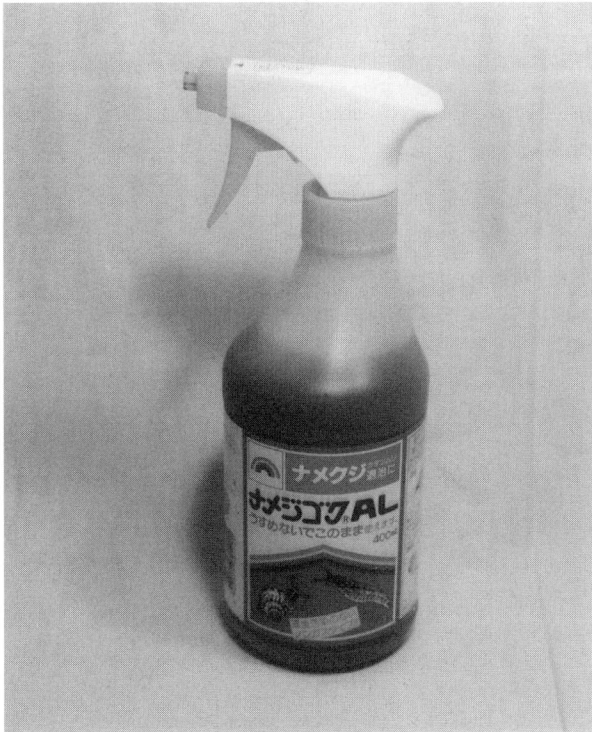

FIG. 33 Slug and snail spray.

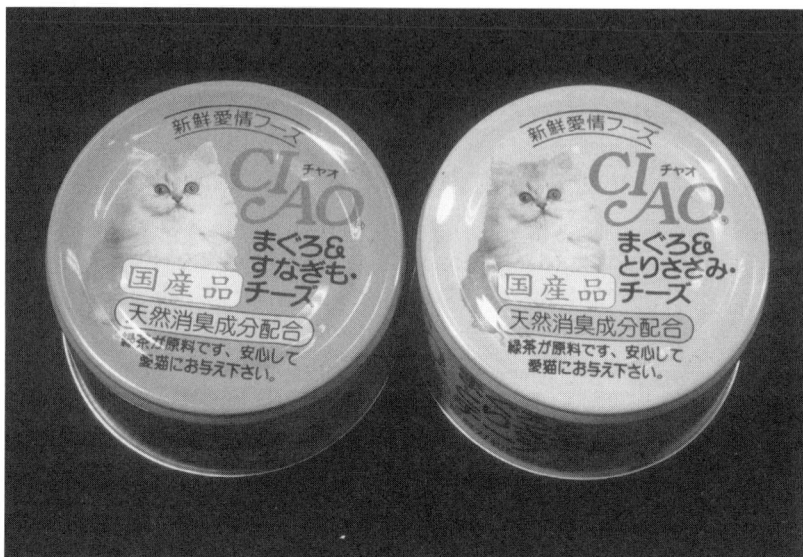

FIG. 34 Cat food enriched with tea catechins.

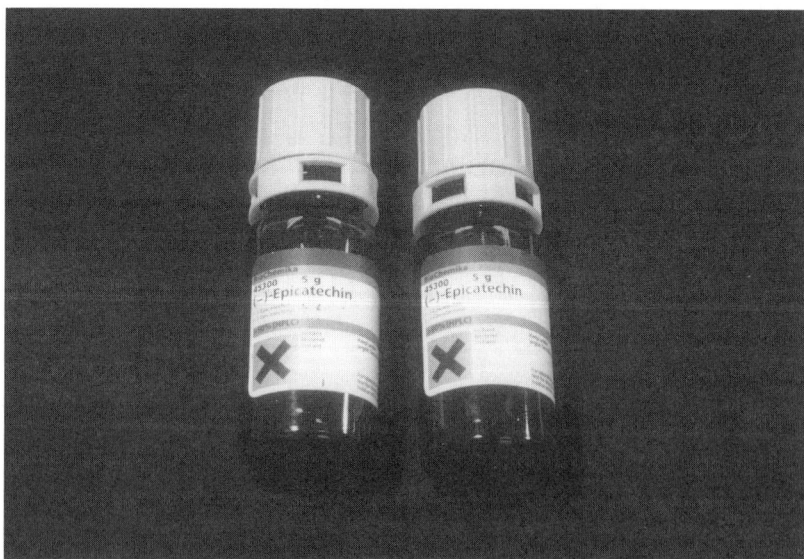

FIG. 35 Pure tea polyphenol compounds.

TABLE 10   Sigma Catalog

Name	Abbreviation
(+)-Catechin	+EC
(−)-Catechin	C
(−)-Epicatechin	EC
(+)-Epicatechin	+EC
(−)-Epigallocatechin	EGC
(−)-Epigallocatechin gallate	EGCg
(−)-Gallocatechin gallate	GCg
(−)-Epicatechin gallate	ECg
(−)-Catechin gallate	Cg
Tea extract (theaflavins)	TFs
Polyphenon-60	P-60
Polyphenon-100	P-100
N-γ-ethyl-L-glutamin (theanine)	—
2-O-β-L-arabinopyranosyl-myo-inositol	—

R. Pure Tea Polyphenol Compounds (Fig. 35)

Pure catechin compounds, a crude mixture of them, and crude theaflavins are distributed by way of Funakoshi Co. in Japan and Sigma Chemical Co. worldwide. Cataloged compounds, as well as those available from Mitsui Norin Co., are listed in Table 10.

20

Tea in Japan

I. TEA PRODUCTION IN JAPAN

A. The Tea Planting Area

The tea planting area of Japan in 1997 was 51,800 ha. This figure is less than 15% of the maximum area of 61,000 ha under production in 1980–1983. In the last five years, there has been an abrupt decrease, and 1000 ha of tea fields are abolished every year. Tea farming is prolific mostly in the southwestern half of the Japanese Archipelago from the Kanto district (where Tokyo is situated) to the southern tip of Kyushu Island. Five prefectures in Japan (Shizuoka, Kagoshima, Mie, Kumamoto, and Kyoto) account for 69% of the area used for tea and Shizuoka Prefecture dominates with 41.3%. Fig. 1 shows the tea planting areas in Japan.

The climatic conditions of the tea growing regions are as follows: average temperature throughout the year is 11.5–

Production of tea in Japan (1998)

Prefecture	Production (tonnes)
Shizuoka	36000
Kagoshima	17000
Mie	6910
Kyoto	3130
Miyazaki	2730
Nara	2380
Fukuoka	2080
Kumamoto	1910
Saga	1730
Saitama	1230
Others	7500
Total	82600

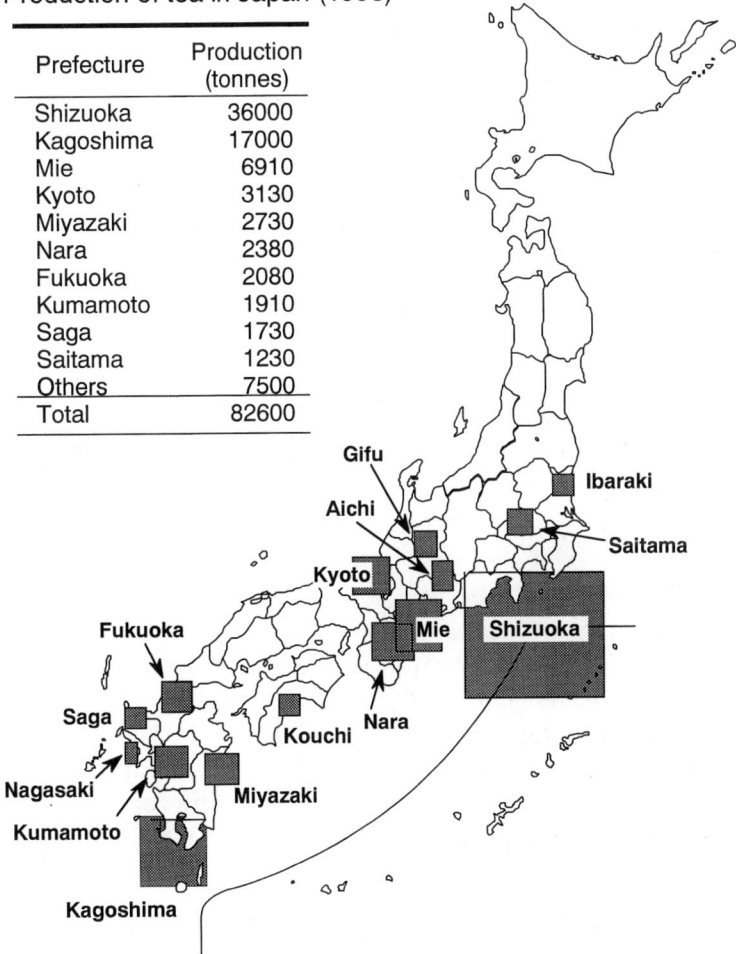

FIG. 1   Green tea production in Japan.

18.0°C; average rainfall is 1500 mm–2000 mm a year. Generally, the yield is higher in the areas where the annual average temperature is above 16°C and it is lower in the areas of under 14°C. Quality tends to show a reverse trend to that of yield in terms of temperature.

B. Production

The total production of tea in Japan in 1998 was about 82,600 tons (tea before sifting and grading). Shizuoka Prefecture dominates in production with about 44% of the total amount of Japanese tea, followed by Kagoshima and Mie Prefectures. It appears that tea fields in mountainous areas and those in suburban areas have decreased and expansion has occurred in those areas where the terrain is flat and large scale mechanical farming is possible. In Table 1 the total planting area and production volume are shown.

C. Varieties

In Japan, almost all teas are made into green tea. In other words, no black tea or oolong tea is made in Japan. The Japanese word for tea is *"cha,"* although it is colloquially called "O'cha," with the honorific "O" preceding it. O'cha is the general word for tea. Among O'cha, *Sen-cha* dominates, accounting for about 75% of total production. The term *Ryoku-cha*, literally "green tea," is usually used to mean Sen-cha. The

TABLE 1 The Total Planting Area and Production of Tea

Year	Planting area (ha)	Production
1970	51,600	77,431
1975	59,200	105,449
1980	61,000	102,300
1985	60,600	95,500
1990	58,500	89,900
1997	51,800	88,700

Chinese characters for Sen-cha literally mean "teas to be brewed," which is the typical way green tea is processed in Japan.

Today, Sen-cha is manufactured in almost every tea district and is available widely in not only shops specializing in tea, but in even the smallest supermarket, making it an integral part of daily life. In the manufacture of Sen-cha, the picked fresh leaves are immediately steamed for 30–40 seconds to inactivate enzymes. After steaming, the leaves are gradually and carefully put through several stages of rolling cum drying to make needle-like shapes.

Following the Sen-cha grades comes *Ban-cha*, which makes up about 14% of total green tea production. Ban-cha is a lower grade of Sen-cha, made from coarse leaves and stalks. "Ban" means literally "grade." Ban-cha possibly denotes "teas out of grades." "Ban" also carries another meaning of "late evening." In this sense, "Ban-cha" could mean the tea made from older leaves or from the late harvest of the year. This variety is losing merit for manufacturers since Ban-cha is considered a cheap tea and is sold in the market as such, in spite of its manufacturing cost. On the other hand, the following three varieties are sold at rather expensive prices: Gyokuro, Kabuse-cha, and Ten-cha.

Gyokuro is the best quality green tea in Japan. The tea plants are cultivated under shade for about two weeks (90% darkness) before harvest. Only the hand-picked soft leaves are used to make this special tea. Production of Gyokuro peaked in 1980 and has been declining since then because of the high price, extra care required for brewing, and changes in the tastes of consumers. *Kabuse-cha* is of good quality, too. The degree and period of shading is shorter (50–80% darkness, 1–2 weeks) than that of Gyokuro. Ten-cha is a kind of shaded tea and is powdered to make *Matcha*, a tea for use in tea ceremony. The sales and uses of this powdered variety are expanding into confectionery and other food markets where it is used to add natural green color and give a distinctive Matcha flavor.

TABLE 2   The Production of Different Varieties of Tea (ton)

Year	Sen-cha	Gyokuro	Kabuse-cha	Ten-cha	Ban-cha	Tama-ryoku-cha	Total
1980	81,300	553	2,450	415	12,100	5,470	102,300
1985	74,700	420	2,950	552	11,500	5,420	92,500
1990	72,700	357	3,180	896	8,020	4,780	89,900
1993	72,200	326	3,250	820	11,100	4,510	92,100
1997	66,600	254	4,090	1,100	9,710	4,250	87,100
1998	61,300	261	4,120	998	7,720	3,700	78,700
Percent	77.8	0.3	5.2	1.3	9.8	4.7	100

In a certain district of Kyushu, a unique round-shaped green tea is manufactured. It is called *Tama-ryoku-cha*, literally "beads-green-tea." In its manufacture, tea leaves are steamed and then rolled vertically in heated drums to give it its characteristic shape and roasted flavor. This tea makes up 5% of the total amount of tea produced. In Table 2 production of different varieties of tea is shown.

Black tea used to be manufactured in Japan, and production peaked at 8225 tons in 1955. After the liberalization of black tea imports in 1972, tropical black teas with their good quality and competitive prices ousted domestic production. Currently, Oolong tea is not produced in Japan, and all of it is imported from China or Taiwan.

II. THE CULTIVATION AND MANUFACTURE OF JAPANESE TEA

In Japan, tea is grown mostly in mountainous areas. About 60% of tea plantations are on hilly ground. The plants are usually planted on the contour. The cross-section of a row of plants is arch shaped with a height of about 60 cm. This is for ease of machine (power) picking. In machine picking, two people proceed along the row of plants holding both ends of the arched power cutter fitted with a loose cotton bag above the surface of the tea. Tea bushes of shaded varieties are grown freely under the shade and picking is done manually.

A. Plant Variety

Until the early 1960s, 90% of the plants were grown from seedlings. Since that time, various clones have been propagated, and today more than 80% of the teas in the main tea districts are clonal. Predominantly, more than 85% of the clones are of the "Yabukita" cultivar. The propagation of the plants is done vegetatively. The cuttings in the nursery are cultivated and are ready to transplant to the tea field after two years. Transplanting is usually done during March and April at a rate of about 18,500 plants per ha.

B. Picking

In the cultivation of the Japanese tea garden, the surface of
the rows of tea are pruned in such a way that the shoots grow
in a regular manner. Very clear seasonal flushing of shoots
and mechanized picking are characteristic of Japanese tea
production and harvest.

Tea used to be harvested two to four times a year, but
three times a year is the recent trend. The first picking is done
during late April to early May for the first flush. The second
picking is done during the middle of June to early July, followed by the third picking in late July to early August. In Sep-
tember or October, there used to be a fourth pick (Autumnal
pick), but it is uncommon now because the leaves do not fetch
a high enough price for the farmers. The first flush in the
springtime has the best quality and farmers get about 80% of
their total yearly revenue from this. The quality declines
sharply in the second or third pick.

Picking is done mostly with a powered picking machine.
Manual picking is only for shaded teas such as Gyokuro or
for limited specialty Sen-cha. The most prevalent picking
machine is a portable type with a power engine which is
operated by two people. This machine picks 60–90 times
more leaves than by hand picking and enables 0.2 ha per
day to be harvested. Lately, in flat areas in Kyushu districts,
the mounted-type picking car is starting to be widely used.
This car picks 1–2 ha per day. In the hilly areas, rail-pickers
are increasingly being used. Rails are put between the
rows and the machine picks the tea while running along the
rails.

C. Fertilizers, Pests, and Diseases

Tea responds to heavy fertilization. In Japan, in order to increase yield and amino acids, nitrogen is used heavily as a
fertilizer (500–800 kg/ha). Phosphate and nitrogen are used
in the ratio of 1:3, and the ratio of potassium to nitrogen is
1:2.

Tea's main pests are: tea leaf rollers, smaller tea tortrix, Oriental tea tortrix, Kanzawa spider mite, and mulberry scale. As far as diseases are concerned, anthracnose (*Collectricum theae-sinensis*) is common. To protect teas from these pests and diseases, agricultural chemicals are allowed under very strict rules and conditions.

D. Climatic Hazards

The most destructive climatic hazard in Japan is frost. From April to early May, when the shoots are about to be picked, tea fields can be devastated by just one frost. In response to past experiences, electric fans have been set up on poles placed throughout the tea fields where frost might occur. From a height of 6 to 8 meters the fan sends slightly warmer air down to the surface to elevate the temperature. An elevation of 2 to 3°C on the tea surface has been confirmed by this method. Alternatively, protection from frosts is sought by covering the shoots with polythene or by sprinkling the plants with water.

E. Manufacture of Green Tea

In the case of Sen-cha, freshly picked leaves have to be steamed as soon as possible to inactivate oxidative enzymes. Mechanized picking has made it possible to scale up the manufacturing plant and hence improve the storage system of the fresh leaves.

Following is the schematic process for Sen-cha production:

Process	Steaming	Primary drying/ rolling	Rolling	Secondary rolling	Final rolling	Drying
Time	30 sec	45 min	20 min	40 min	40 min	30 min
Temperature used	100°C	95°C	Room temperature	34°C Exhaust air	90°C	80°C
Temperature of leaves	98°C	35°C	Room temperature	36°C	40°C	70 °C
Weight	100%	45%	—	30%	25%	23%

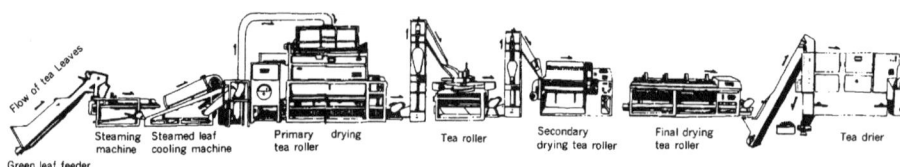

FIG. 2 Manufacture of green tea.

In accordance with the amount to be processed in one batch, there are several systems, from the 35K series which has a capacity of 30 kg of fresh leaves to the 240K series which has a capacity of 200 kg of fresh leaves. In recent popular systems, all the above processes are designed to work automatically, as shown in Fig. 2. Teas thus made in the cooperative factories are called "Ara-cha" or "crude tea."

F. Processing of Crude Tea for the Market

Crude teas made in the cooperative factories have to be further processed or refined for retail packaging. Crude teas from various origins are bought and stocked in the refrigerated godowns of processing factories. The lots chosen for blending are refired (dried) to give longer shelf life and better flavor. After re-drying, each crude tea will be sifted and graded according to size. Finally, each lot will be blended according to the blend order by the tasters and be packed for sale.

G. Storage

Green tea is more sensitive to deterioration by heat or moisture than black tea or oolong tea. In order to increase shelf life, it is essential to reduce the moisture content to 2–3% in the above refiring process. Teas should be packaged in moisture-proof containers. With certain brands, the air in the package is replaced by nitrogen gas to protect the tea from oxidative deterioration. It is recommended that packaged teas bought at the store should be kept under dark conditions at 05°C, usually in the refrigerator, until use.

III. THE PROCESSING AND CONSUMPTION OF TEA IN JAPAN

All Japanese teas are cultivated by individual farmers (small holders). In 1996, there were 307,300 households in Japan cultivating tea. Only about 10% of these small holders cultivated more than 1 ha (ca. 2.5 acres). The average acreage for one household is 0.29 ha. Tea leaves picked by these farmers are carried by cargo lorries to the factory. There are three kinds of factories:

1. A farmer's own factory,
2. A cooperative factory run by several farmers together
3. A factory that buys tea leaves

Recently, big scale cooperative factories run by a group of farmers are increasing. Teas thus processed and dried are put in 60 kg paper bags as crude tea. These crude teas are sold to the processing factories that are located nearer the city, and where refiring, sifting, grading, blending, and packaging are done for the market. A fairly large amount of crude tea can be kept for months in the huge refrigerated go-downs before packaging. The first flush tea of the May pick is dominant in volume and far superior in quality and price than the second flush teas of July. Therefore, the first flush teas are kept for blending until the next new season. Tea quality is well preserved at 0–5°C but deteriorates at higher temperatures. Because of the vulnerability of Sen-cha in storage, the amount in a package for sale is usually 100 g or 200 g. The amount purchased per household (family) was 2325 g a year (529 g per head) in 1972. The figure decreased to 1242 g per family (352 g per head) in 1996. The reasons for this decline are ascribed to the Westernization of daily foods and to heavy competition with other beverages. The older generation tends to buy more green tea than the younger generation. The most popular price range seems to be U.S. $5–10 per 100 g. In recent years, in line with the convenience-oriented lifestyle that has become prevalent these days, the ready-to-drink sector of the market has come into its own with a surge in demand for canned or bottled green teas.

IV. THE IMPORT AND EXPORT OF TEA IN JAPAN

A. Export

There was a time when Japanese green tea enjoyed booming exports. The peak was in 1917, when about 80% of the green tea produced in Japan was exported to the United States During the Pacific War (1941–1945) there were no exports. Following the war, in the 1950s to 1960s, green tea exports were resumed to North African countries, such as Morocco, at a rate as high as 17,000 tons/year at a time. Exports declined from the 1970s onward and are at present minimal. This decline of Japanese tea exports might be ascribed to the following reasons: (a) people in the United States preferred black tea to green tea, and (b) Japanese green tea is more expensive than teas from other sources. Recently, however, it is likely that Japanese green tea might again find a place in the global market, since people in Europe and the United States are becoming aware of the health benefits and are showing interest in Japanese green tea.

B. Imports

With improvements in the standard of living over the last decades, imports of black tea, oolong tea, and green tea have increased markedly as shown in Fig. 3. One of the reasons for this abrupt increase in tea imports in recent years is related to consumers' desire for convenience in their daily lives. People today prefer canned or bottled ready-to-drink (RTD) teas to the teas that have to be brewed at home. There are countless vending machines and numerous convenience stores in every town. People buy canned or bottled RTD teas at these facilities. Industrially, the canning of black tea started first,

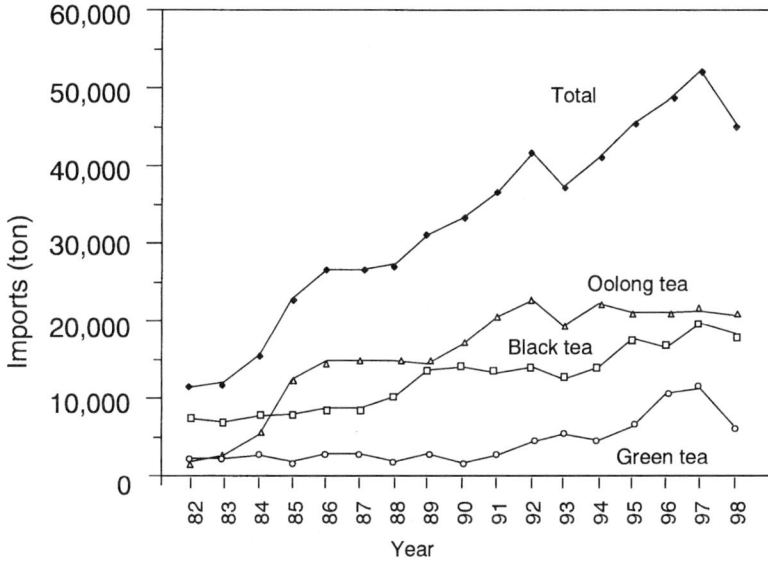

FIG. 3   Recent trends in tea import.

followed by oolong tea. Green tea consumers have been and still are reluctant to shift from home brew to bottled tea. In any case, trends in the import of various teas parallel those of the volume of RTD teas. Black tea is mostly and almost equally imported from India and Sri Lanka. Oolong tea is imported predominantly from China with marginal tons from Taiwan.

Green tea from abroad found a niche in the Japanese market around 1970, when it began to be used in blending. In 1973 as much as 12,800 tons of green tea, mainly from Taiwan, were imported into Japan. They were used for fillers in the lower grade varieties but gradually the volume declined to 1941 tons in 1990 because Japanese people preferred better quality teas at a higher price to cheaper, more pungent teas. Recently, the picture seems to have changed and imports of green tea have begun to increase, reaching 10,824 tons in 1996. This trend is likely to continue increase steadily. Although the green tea market has diversified in RTD and many other uses, and the demand for middle to lower grade teas is increasing, Japanese green tea production could not possibly fill demand, particularly for the lower grade teas. There is no incentive for Japanese farmers to harvest lower grade teas which are unprofitable. The main countries exporting green tea to Japan are China, Taiwan, Vietnam, Brazil, Indonesia, Bangladesh, and New Zealand. Among them, China dominates with 73% of the total import figure.

V. RECENT TRENDS IN THE JAPANESE TEA INDUSTRY

Over the last 15 years, with the advent of vending machines, convenience stores and the easy availability of cars to everybody, the ready-to drink soft drinks are gaining in growing popularity among the convenience-oriented, mobile young generations throughout the country. Accordingly the consumption of canned (bottled) teas are growing as shown in Fig. 4. In recent years, in the ready-to-drink (RTD) tea sector, combinations of teas with those of herbal origins have been gaining in remarkable popularity. In 1993, a product known as "16 Varieties of Tea" made from extracted green tea mixed with 15 kinds of herbs was bottled and sold by Asahi Brewery. This original product gained acceptance with the consumers and the marketing of various such mixed tea drinks followed suit, thus establishing such beverages consisting of tea/herb mixtures as one of the main categories in bottled tea drinks. Inclusive of these varieties, the production trends of "tea drinks" as compared with those of other soft drinks are shown in Fig. 5. As it is clear from the figure, the growth of tea drinks over the last ten years and their future potential is phenomenal; whereas the market for carbonated drinks, which was once dominant, as well as that of fruit juices and coffee drinks, which was at one time growing, are now both saturated. The

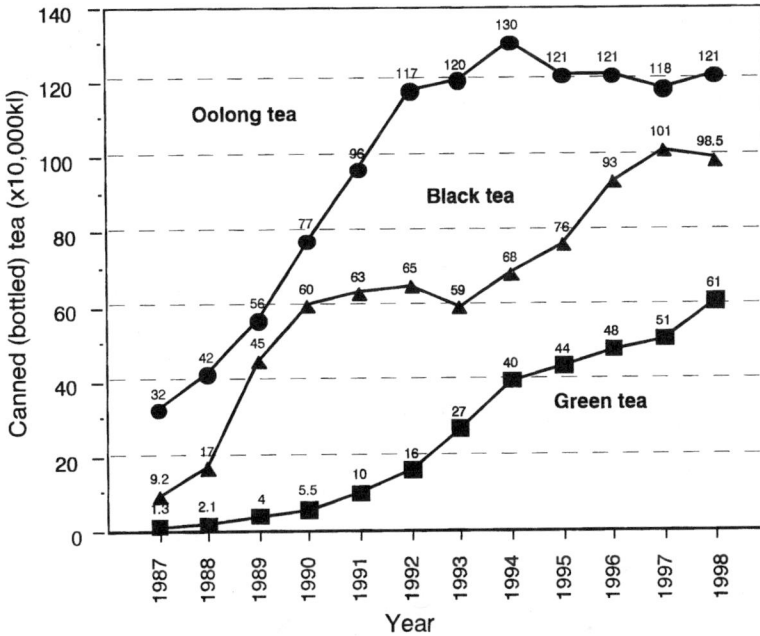

FIG. 4   Trends in consumption of canned tea.

reason for this extraordinary growth of tea drinks is ascribed primarily to the consumers' recognition of the health benefits of tea, backed up perhaps by improved techniques in producing tea drinks with good flavors.

A.   The Vending Machine Market

During the 1980s, the vending machine market developed markedly, and operators deployed machines throughout the country. The system in Japan is that the operators buy both the machine and the canned products, and find a tenant to install the machine. The routemen deliver the cans, maintain the machine, and collect the money deposited. Cola and a variety of canned coffees have been the main merchandise in this expanding vending machine market. In Japan, both tea and

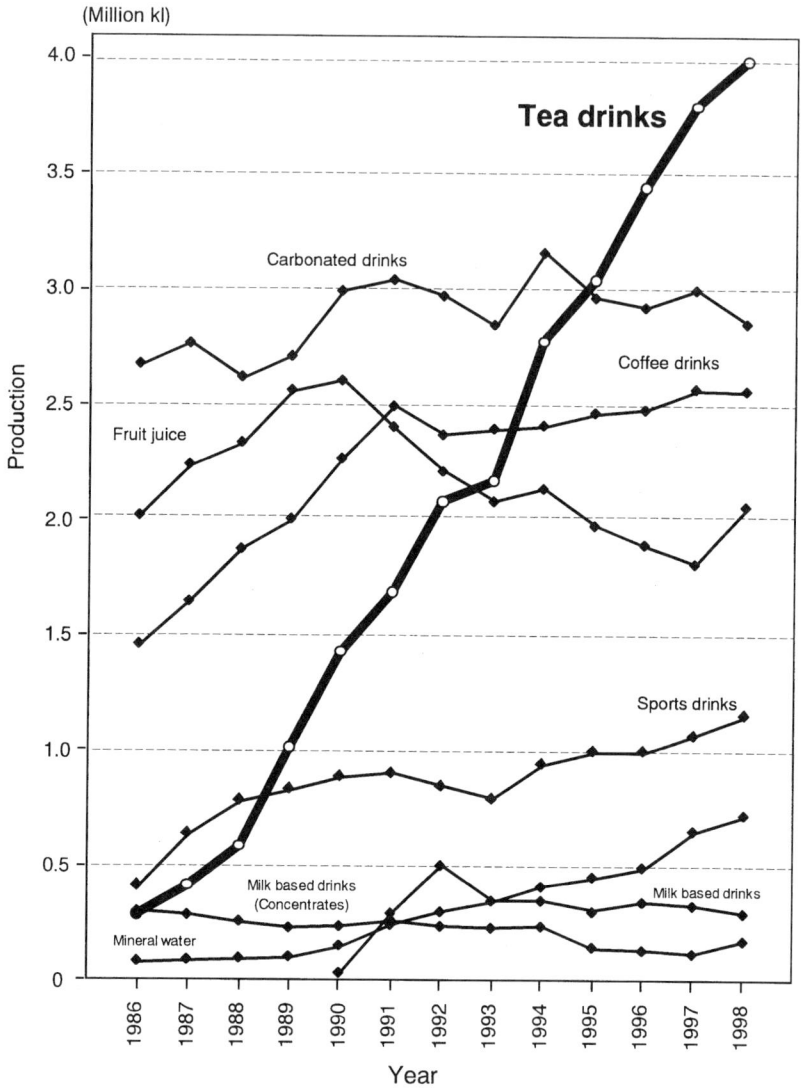

FIG. 5 Trends in production of various soft drinks in Japan.

coffee are sold hot in winter and cold in summer from vending machines, creating a selling advantage over cola and other soft drinks, which are only consumed cold. Presently there are 2.5 million vending machines in operation for soft drinks. In 1998 more than 69% of the total canned soft drink products were sold through vending machines, as compared with 31% from supermarket outlets.

B. Production of Black Tea Beverages

Black tea beverages in the form of soft drinks were first marketed in Japan in 1973 by Pokka Corporation. They were lemon flavored, sweetened with sugar, and packed in 250 ml steel cans. A year later, Mitsui Norin Company entered the market selling cans of three different sugar-sweetened flavors: lemon, milk, and brandy. Production of these black tea beverages remained rather constant in the following 10 years, that is, roughly 2 million cases a year (250 ml × 30 cans/case) were sold. During this period, a dramatic increase in sales of canned coffee beverages was recorded. In 1984 companies that produced widely consumed beverage brands joined the market with lemon or milk tea, and the market expanded to 10 million cases a year within a few years. Varieties in packaging and volume sizes were introduced, for example, aluminum or steel cans (190, 250, and 340 grams), paper, plastic (PET) bottles, glass bottles, etc. In 1988 Kirin Brewery Company (the largest brewery in Japan) entered the market with plain-type teas (no fruit flavors, with or without milk, little or no sugar) under the brand name Afternoon Tea. Emphasis was laid on the fact that these teas contained minimum or no sugar, attracting the attention of health-conscious consumers. This brand alone sold more than 300 million cases a year (340 g × 24/case equivalent). In 1990 nearly 8000 tons, or more than 50% of total black tea imports were extracted, not in homes, but in factories. It was estimated that the volume of canned black tea for beverage packs would exceed about 100 million cases in 1999. Production processes of canned tea (plain, lemon, and milk) are summarized in Fig. 6.

C. Production of Oolong Tea Beverages

Canned oolong tea was pioneered by Ito-en Company in 1981. At that time, other canned products contained sweeteners. Oolong tea, with its herbal appeal, was preferred by young women because of its noncaloric nature, and it was also advertised for men as a chaser after consumption of alcoholic drinks. In 1993 more than 100 million cases were sold. In this category, Suntory Company shares more than one third of the total can and PET bottle market, followed by Coca Cola Company, the Kirin and Asahi Breweries, Pokka, Ito-en, and many other companies.

Oolong tea is consumed plain, without any additives. The production of canned oolong tea is thus straightforward because there is no necessity for quality control for additives as in the case of lemon or milk teas.

D. Production of Green Tea Beverages

The Japanese green tea industry has been self-sufficient and has not been exposed to any fierce competition from outside. However, because the flavor of green tea is so ingrained on Japanese palates, the production of canned green tea is very difficult. Many attempts have been made to bottle or can green tea in a way that will appeal to the general Japanese public. Older generations, who are often bound by traditional ideas about green tea drinking, find it difficult to adjust to the flavor of canned green tea, which must be subjected to high temperatures in order to ensure safety in storage. Only over the last few years has canned green tea gained popular recognition with substantial selling volume.

Although green tea is consumed plain, with no extra additives, the canning process must be carried out with utmost care because canned green tea is very susceptible to high temperatures in the sterilization process and to oxidation during

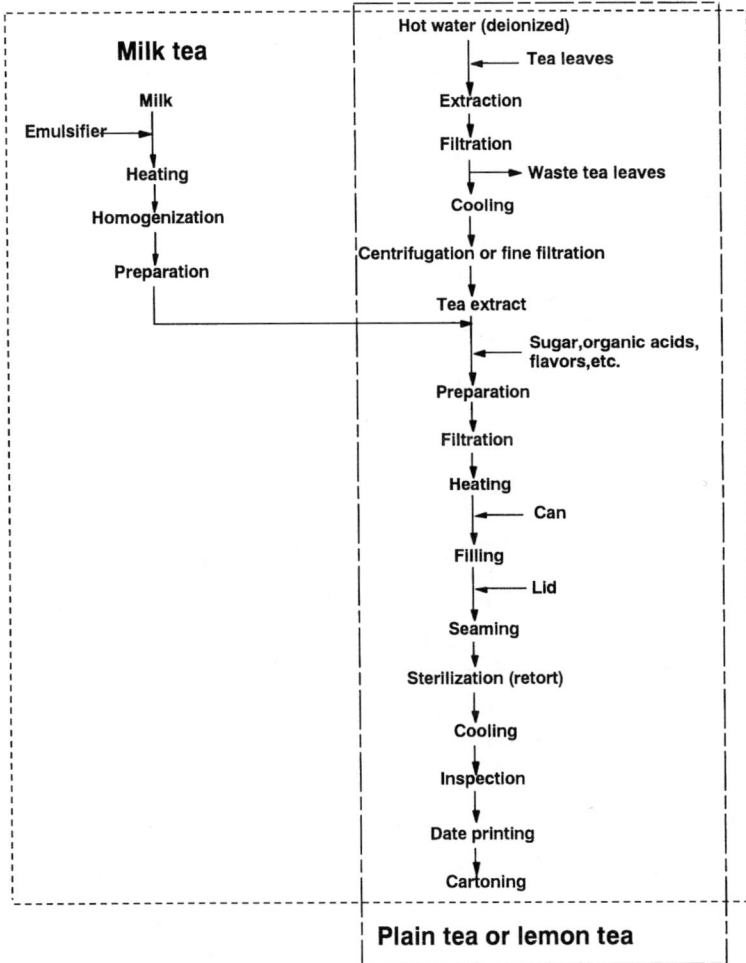

FIG. 6 The canned tea production process.

storage, factors which cause color deterioration over time. Usually, to prevent oxidation, vitamin C is added, and the headspace air is replaced with nitrogen.

Section IV presents the details of the canned tea production process and the necessary quality controls for each ingredient.

VI. TECHNOLOGY OF CANNED TEA PRODUCTION

A. Facilities and the Production Process

1. Production Facility

The canning or bottling factory should follow the codes of good manufacturing practice (GMP). The following is an example of the production process, of which there may be variations.

2. Extraction and Filtration

Extraction of tea is conducted with extraction machines specifically designed for tea. Waste tea leaves are automatically removed. Fibrous residues remain in the extracted solution. These fluffy residues of tea leaves are removed by paper or cloth filtration. This filtration prevents latent sedimentation in storage of the end product. The preparation is further filtered to clarify the liquid.

3. Pasteurization

The preparation is pasteurized by passing it through a plate heater under predetermined conditions. In the ultra high temperature (UHT) system, plain tea or lemon tea is pasteurized at 135°C for 15 seconds. These conditions exceed those necessary for bactericidal effect, i.e., 4 minutes at 121°C, to sterilize the spores of *Clostridium botulinum*. These conditions can be adjusted to 3 seconds at 110°C if no milk is involved in the preparation.

4. Filling, Seaming, and Cooling

Filling temperature of the preparation should be around 80–90°C. The pasteurized preparation, which is at a higher temperature, cools to these levels while traveling in the tube from the plate heater to the filling tank by way of a surge tank. After seaming the lid, the can should be cooled as soon as possible. Usually, cans are cooled to normal temperature while traveling through a water-spraying tunnel.

5. Inspection and Packaging

The weight and the seaming are inspected automatically on the assembly line to ensure proper filling and hermetic sealing. Then the date of production is printed on the base of the can, and the cans are transported on a conveyor belt to a packaging machine where they are placed in cartons for storage and shipping.

B. Ingredients

1. Water

Water should be chlorinated or ultraviolet (UV) irradiated to sterilize any bacterial infection which may be present; then it should be dechlorinated by active carbon. The water should also be deionized to remove all metallic ions.

2. Tea Leaves

In selecting a tea in blending teas for extraction, the first consideration should be its quality as a normal brew, that is, a good flavor and a good liquid color. Secondly, the brew should have little cream (complex of polyphenols and caffeine) on cooling. Usually quality tea has more cream than mediocre tea, but the ideal is to find a good tea without heavy creaming. When cream is unavoidable, tannase treatment should be applied to the extracted liquid (0.25% of tannase [500 units/g] of soluble solids) so that the esterified polyphenols which tend to form cream are decomposed into less cream forming simple polyphenols and gallic acid.

3. Sugar

Usually isomerized liquid sugar from a sugar refinery is used and stored in a tank in the factory. This liquid sugar is produced by the isomerization of glucose into fructose by isomerase treatment. At one point in the conveying tube on the way to the preparation tank, the liquid sugar is sterilized by UV irradiation. When crystallized sucrose is dissolved directly into the preparation tank, utmost care should be taken to avoid infection of the sugar during storage.

4. Organic Acids

Usually citric acid is used to supplement the acidity of lemon tea, in place of or in addition to filtered, concentrated lemon juice. In certain cases, a trace of ascorbic acid (vitamin C) may be added to prevent the oxidative deterioration of the product before consumption.

5. Flavors

Heat tolerance of the flavors must be analyzed experimentally prior to the actual production. In order to preserve the good flavors of tea or lemon, extreme heating should be avoided in the sterilization process.

6. Milk

Contamination-free milk is a prerequisite. Pasteurized milk should be stored in a tank specifically cooled for this purpose. When powdered milk is used, it should be dissolved in hot water separately in a special tank before it is pumped into the preparation tank.

7. Head Space

Replacement of head space air of the can with nitrogen is recommended. Filling with the tea preparations at high temperatures (about 85°C) will render the pressure of the can negative (40–50 mmHg) on cooling.

8. Cans and Lids

Prior to filling, the empty cans should be washed with chlorinated water, and the residual water should be removed by putting them upside down of the feeding rail. Immediately after the can is filled with the hot preparation, the lid is seamed automatically. After seaming, the can is turned upside down so that the lid is sterilized by the heat.

VII. SUMMARY

The present situation and prospects for tea production is rather gloomy. Small holders presently engaged in tea farming are getting older and in many tea districts nearly 50% of farmers are over 65 years old. Moreover, in most of these households, there are no young people willing to take on farming as their livelihood, and thus a decline in productivity and an increase in the number of desolate tea fields is proceeding at a rapid pace. In order to cope with this situation, the authorities are encouraging farmers to scale up their fields by integrating deserted lots as well as introducing cooperative or mandatory management of several lots. In addition, in order to offer more incentives to farmers, investments in such areas as mechanization in farming and factory automation are being subsidized. Still, problems remain, particularly in the tea fields in mountainous areas. In these areas, the fields are small and incorporation of lots is geographically difficult. Further, these areas are remote, making access and transportation difficult. Working on hilly slopes is hard and the yield is low. There is also the problem of soil erosion and difficult climatic conditions. It is certain that tea fields in hilly districts will be abandoned at a much faster pace.

The outlook for tea consumption, however, seems to be rather rosy. The health benefits of green tea are gaining national recognition. In addition to the drinking of tea, wider

applications for tea and its components are being discovered.
Tea's antioxidative, antibacterial, deodorant, and other properties are being put to use in various ways. The total consumption of green tea remains level, although the demand for tea
for use in tea bags or for ready-to-drink products is increasing.
Competition with other beverages is still severe in these expanding sectors.

In the future, the Japanese green tea industry should ef-
ficiently produce high-quality, more expensive teas in suitable
areas, and aim at pleasing the discerning tastes of people. On
the other hand, middle to low grade teas for RTD drinks or
for other nondrinking uses will be in greater demand. There
is no other way but to import these grades of green teas from
abroad. In 1996, total tea imports were 48,420 tons a year.
This figure is about half that of total domestic production.
Among these imports, about 77.6% is composed of oolong tea
and black tea combined, the rest being green tea. The percentage of imports that green tea holds will grow in the future.

With the growing recognition of the health benefits of
green tea in the United States and in European countries
where people are health conscious, the export of Japanese tea
is likely to increase. To answer this demand, good quality, rea-
sonably priced Japanese teas should be produced, which will
be attractive to people in developed countries. In Japan, too,
the concern for organic farming in general, and the demand
for nonchemical, organically grown teas in particular, is increasing. At the same time, people today tend to prefer characteristic products to mass produced ones.

Taking all the above trends into account, the basic direc-
tion for the future of the tea industry in Japan is to produce
high quality teas or characteristically outstanding teas, aim-
ing primarily at domestic consumption.

Index